PRESCRIPTION FOR LONGEVITY

Other books by James Scala

Making the Vitamin Connection
The Arthritis Relief Diet
The High Blood Pressure Relief Diet
Eating Right for a Bad Gut

By James Scala and Barbara Jacques

Look 10 Years Younger, Feel 10 Years Better

PRESCRIPTION FOR LONGEVITY

EATING RIGHT FOR A LONG LIFE

DR. JAMES SCALA

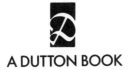

A DUTTON BOOK

DUTTON
Published by the Penguin Group
Penguin Books USA Inc., 375 Hudson Street,
New York, New York 10014, U.S.A.
Penguin Books Ltd, 27 Wrights Lane,
London W8 5TZ, England
Penguin Books Australia Ltd, Ringwood,
Victoria, Australia
Penguin Books Canada Ltd, 10 Alcorn Avenue,
Toronto, Ontario, Canada M4V 3B2
Penguin Books (N.Z.) Ltd, 182-190 Wairau Road,
Auckland 10, New Zealand

Penguin Books Ltd, Registered Offices:
Harmondsworth, Middlesex, England

First published by Dutton, an imprint of New American Library,
a division of Penguin Books USA Inc.
Distributed in Canada by McClelland & Stewart Inc.

First Printing, March, 1992
10 9 8 7 6 5 4 3 2 1

  REGISTERED TRADEMARK—MARCA REGISTRADA

LIBRARY OF CONGRESS CATALOGING-IN-PUBLICATION DATA:
Scala, James, 1934–
    Prescription for longevity : eating right for a long life / James Scala.
        p.   cm.
Includes bibliographical references and index.
ISBN 0-525-93413-8
1. Nutrition   2. Longevity.   I. Title.
RA784.S378   1992
613.2—dc20   91-32456
                                                                      CIP

Printed in the United States of America
Set in Times Roman
Designed by Leonard Telesca

NOTE TO THE READER
The ideas, procedures, and suggestions contained in this book are not intended as a substitute
for consulting with your physician. All matters regarding your health require medical supervision.

Our parents, Louis and Lorene, Warren and Ethel:

Children are living messages that we send to
  a time we will not see.

This book is yours.

—Jim and Nancy

Contents

Acknowledgments   ix
Disclaimer   xi
Preface   xiii
Introduction: The Protectors   1

I. ANTIOXIDANTS   15

1. Beta Carotene and Carotenoids   17
2. Vitamin C   40
3. Vitamin E and Tocopherols   65
4. Selenium   87
5. Taurine   97

II. REGULATORS   109

   6. Fiber   111
   7. Protective Fiber in Food   132
   8. Balancing Essential Oils   148
   9. Gamma Linolenic Acid   173
  10. Folic Acid   181
  11. Niacin   194
  12. Calcium and Sunshine   200

III. PROTECTOR FOODS   215

  13. Garlic, Onions, Leeks, and Shallots Too   217
  14. Cruciferous Vegetables   233

IV. THE LONGEVITY PROGRAM   243

  15. The Longevity Diet: Don't Get Older, Get Better 245
  16. The Longevity Diet Menus: One Day at a Time   259

APPENDIX   277

Additional Reading   279
Index   287

Acknowledgments

Nancy: When you said, "for better or worse," you didn't know it included lunch. Thanks for your typing, research, editing, and most of all your smile.

Alexia Dorszynski: Thanks for getting behind all my ideas and for gently injecting your excellent knowledge.

Kristin Olson: I look forward to watching your star rise.

Al Zuckerman: Thanks for getting behind the idea and suffering through the preliminaries.

Jon Price: Thanks for your suggestions, ideas, and encouragement.

Nan and Kim: For the late meals, long discussions, hours when Mom and I were working; your support was important and appreciated.

Ilene Storace: Thanks for your help with my many literature searches.

Alice Tramontana of McCormick & Co., Inc., R&D Labs: For help in my garlic quest.

Pat Najarian: Thanks for reading and critiquing the complete text.

Disclaimer

This book is about personal responsibility. It contains a simple message: "There are things in food that help protect and preserve your health." It also contains positive advice on steps you can take to preserve your health and extend your life.

However, this book is no substitute for your doctor. If you get sick, you should see a physician. Indeed, I recommend having an annual examination, even if you feel great. Modern medicine works miracles, and not to use its incredible power is foolish, but it's still a poor substitute for prevention.

Prevention will always be the best medicine. Prevention is a personal responsibility that can only be practiced by you. Governments can require vaccines and inoculations to prevent obvious diseases, but they can't legislate what you eat; worse yet, what you don't eat. That's up to you. You can learn about the protectors from this book, but how you apply this information is up to you. You can make this knowledge work for you by eating correctly, exercising regularly, and developing a good lifestyle where you live, work, and play. By example, you will instill these habits in your children and make their lives more abundant.

LIVING LONGER: LIVING BETTER

By applying the knowledge in this book, and taking advantage of modern medicine, you can add over 30 percent to your years. However, the knowledge is worthless if you don't apply it every day of your life. Illness never takes a holiday and neither does good health. Since medicine will continue to advance, the 30-percent extension of life may really be 50 percent or more. But medicine will always favor those who are well. Therefore, our health will always be in our hands, and prevention will reign supreme.

Preface

OUR MODERN EPIDEMIC

If we could prevent all deaths before age fifty, our present life expectancy of seventy-eight years would only increase by about three or four years. In 1900 our life expectancy wasn't fifty years. Since then, we've eliminated most infections and diseases that killed a great many people before age fifty. However, we are now faced with some new challenges to life we call degenerative diseases. They include heart disease, cancer, and stroke. We're making much headway on heart disease and stroke, but cancer is rapidly becoming enemy number one!

Degenerative implies that these diseases develop from age. Sure, our bodies decline with age, but there's no reason the majority of us need to get cancer or heart disease. It might do us better to name these challenges "the preventable diseases." Think of them that way and the concepts in this book can give you a new perspective.

PREVENTION: THE GOAL

Over 60 percent of all deaths are diet-related. This means that over five people in America die every two minutes from an illness that eating correctly could have either prevented completely or put far off into the future. Therefore, selecting the correct foods can pay big dividends.

This high level of diet-related diseases doesn't square with the miraculous possibilities of modern medicine. It doesn't seem right that we can routinely transplant kidneys, repair hearts, keep premature babies alive, and not eat correctly. It's as if we're geniuses in one respect and idiots in the other.

Protector is the name I give to some materials in food that reduce your risk of illness. Protector materials are obtained from food and can even be the food itself, but they have no official nutritional status. This raises a question: Should protectors be given official recognition? I want you to answer that question as you read this book. Some protectors boost our immune system, our main line of defense. Other protectors neutralize toxins that are everywhere in our complex world. In these ways, the protectors prevent major illnesses, such as cancer, and minor disorders, such as stomach discomfort. Together they can all add years to your life and life to your years.

If you're an average woman, your odds of getting breast cancer are one in ten. These odds can be decreased by 20 percent with a diet that provides 320 milligrams of vitamin C, five times the recommended daily allowance. How much vitamin C will you aim for? Will you take a vitamin C supplement? A 20-percent return is excellent by any standards.

Just over seventeen new cases of colorectal cancer appear every hour. In the same hour, seven people die from colorectal cancer. Major risks for these cancers are heredity, polyps, a high-fat, low-fiber diet, in addition to bowel disorders. All of the risks, except heredity, can be reduced by the correct fiber, carotenoids, some specific vegetables, and other nutrients. I want this new knowledge to influence your eating habits.

Most colorectal cancer is diagnosed around age fifty-five, when you're at your peak of productivity. For example, it's the age at which surgeons are usually most skillful, lawyers earn their most money, and executives get promoted. For seventeen people every hour, that productivity comes to an abrupt halt. If you follow the concepts in this book, you'll reduce your risk of colorectal cancer by over 30 percent.

Gallstones and gall-bladder problems have become so prevalent that some hospitals take out full-page ads extolling the ease of their gall-bladder surgery. One regular ad says that four hundred thousand such operations are performed annually in the United States. That's over forty-five every hour! If you reduce these statistics by 50 percent for typical advertising puffery, that's still twenty-three gall-bladder surgeries per hour in the United States. Most gall-bladder problems can be prevented by the right protector foods. Will you use this knowledge to change your eating habits if they're wrong or reinforce them if they're already correct?

Heart disease causes 36 percent of all deaths in the United States. Stroke, a very close relative, accounts for about 10 percent more deaths. Together they account for over three deaths every two minutes. So, add the 22 percent from cancer and we've accounted for over 68 percent of all deaths. Each of these killers is extensively diet-related, so prevention is largely in our own hands.

A low-fat, low-cholesterol, high-fiber diet is essential to reduce the risk of heart disease and stroke. The same dietary program reduces the risk of cancer and many other diseases. If you follow the Longevity Diet in this book to get more protectors, you will reduce your risk of heart disease. By exercising regularly and practicing weight control, you'll greatly improve the quality of your life.

At this point you might ask, "How do I get these protectors or where is this diet?"

The answers to these questions are in this book. After we discuss the major protectors, you'll see how easily they fit into a plan I call the "Longevity Diet." This plan exceeds the surgeon general's program to reduce heart disease and will assure you of getting a basic level of the protectors, which will dramatically reduce your risk of cancer. However, I hope you will opt for more of some protectors by going beyond the plan and using supplements.

LONGEVITY DIET: WHEN DO I START?

Anyone at any age can follow the Longevity Diet because it's not rigid and encourages you to eat many foods. As you read this book, you will realize that by adding more fruits, vegetables, and cereals to your diet, you'll be getting more of the protectors. Alternatively, the same food technology that fills supermarket shelves with junk food, fast food, and processed foods also makes food supplements easily available. Although some experts will say supplements are a waste of money, once you've read a few chapters in this book, you'll ask, ''Compared to what?'' You'll be able to make an informed decision, and unless you're very unusual, you will change your food and food-supplement habits for the better.

PRESCRIPTION FOR LONGEVITY

INTRODUCTION

The Protectors

AN EXCITING DISCOVERY

Brussels sprouts protect us from lung cancer, carrots are good for our eyes, and fish is brain food. Do you dismiss these comments and other old wives' tales as unscientific? After all, they seem unsophisticated and overly simplistic in a world of computers, CAT scans, and magnetic imaging technology. However, if a scientist from Harvard Medical School says that carotenoids protect you from lung cancer, do you want to know where to get them? If that scientist then says, "Eat broccoli regularly," what vegetable are you going to order with dinner?

Suppose another scientist, a physician from Chiba Medical School in Japan, says that the oil DHA is important for healthy brain and eye tissue in adults and absolutely essential for the proper development of these tissues in infants. Then he says that DHA is passed to the infant through mother's milk. When he says you get DHA from oily fish, such as salmon, what will you look for on the menu? What food will you favor if you're nursing?

We all want to be healthy, live a long life, and quietly drift into eternal sleep at the end. Many things make this ideal possible. Modern medicine can go a long way toward getting us well, but the high-tech methods of today's medical practices and the side effects of drugs are scary, sometimes deadly, and often worse than

1

the disease they're used against. So prevention is still the best medicine. In the last ten years, scientists have discovered substances that can extend your life and improve its quality. What makes these substances so exciting is their protective or preventive qualities, so I call them ''protectors.'' Now we can eat foods rich in protectors to prevent specific diseases—and food doesn't have the negative side effects that high-tech medicines do. Since we've got to eat, why not select foods that give us the best protection from illness?

As for living a long life, the average life expectancy has passed the biblical forecast of three score and ten (seventy years) and is within sight of the one hundred and twenty-five to one hundred and fifty years that biologists predict. By preventing cancer and following the surgeon general's advice on heart disease and high blood pressure, you can increase your life expectancy by 30 percent. Think of what that means. If you're about thirty years old and your career is just beginning, treat it as your first, because you'll be able to have two careers with over twenty years in each and still have a nice long retirement. Your children can have three careers with a twenty-year retirement. You just have to protect your health and focus your attention on things that increase the quality of your years.

We now know what causes vitamin deficiencies and most infectious diseases, and we can prevent many of them. Surgery routinely performs miracles to correct what cannot be or was not prevented. Heart disease is understood, and by meeting the AIDS challenge, we'll learn how to conquer viruses. What, then, stands in the way of our being disease-free? We'll always need to protect ourselves from the diseases that result from environmental damage to our body. Now that we're living longer, the things that detract from health have longer to work their havoc on us. That's where the protectors come in: they're our first line of defense.

WHAT DO THEY DO?

The protectors shield us from invisible hazards in life. Some of them neutralize the ultraviolet light from the sun and prevent skin cancer and colon cancer. Others neutralize toxic agents that either directly or indirectly create flaws in the body's first line of defense, the quality of its membranes. The membranes that line the lungs, the digestive tract, and the excretory and reproductive organs are especially susceptible to cancer and permanent damage, as is the case with emphysema.

Some protectors work in concert with other nutrients to shore up the immune system. When these protectors are in the right balance, they help to moderate inflammation and reduce the risk of inflammatory diseases, such as arthritis, and even some forms of migraine headache. In these diseases the immune system has gone awry and attacks its own tissues because the essential balance among some protectors has not been maintained—most people don't eat the correct foods to keep up that balance.

It's not only dramatic diseases, such as cancer or arthritis, that we're dealing with. A few of the protectors simply help us sleep more soundly and think more clearly. The protectors are substances we get from food. If we eat a little more carefully, we'll get enough when we need them most.

ARE THEY VITAMINS?

A few of the protectors are vitamins, and one, beta carotene, is used by our body to make vitamin A. But when a vitamin is also a protector, its protector role is different from its vitamin role, and the amounts needed for each role are different. Scientists and doctors have known about some protectors for a long time, but only in the last decade, and especially in the last few years, have their protector roles been understood. I'll let you decide if they should be designated by the government as "required nutrients," like vitamins.

The role of vitamins was discovered when scientists found that a variety of illnesses resulted from the lack of a particular vitamin in the diet. Vitamin B_1, for example, was identified by chemists who extracted it from foods, such as rice hulls, and gave it to people with deficiency symptoms. Vitamin B_1, or thiamine, deficiency starts with mental depression, progresses to diarrhea, is followed by severe skin disorders, and can end in death. By restoring vitamin B_1 at any stage, except very near death, the doctors stopped the progression of the disease, reversed the symptoms, and returned their patients to satisfactory health.

In contrast to the illnesses caused by vitamin deficiencies, the illnesses that protectors help us avoid aren't generally thought of as deficiencies. However, scientific papers are beginning to appear that make reference to deficiencies of some of these protector materials, especially two, taurine (an unusual amino acid) and EPA (fish oil). Children are so healthy nowadays that we can identify the subtle developmental flaws that emerge from a lack of either one of these two protectors. These developmental problems are so rare that most new cases are written up in medical journals. If caught early enough, the flaw can even be reversed.

VITAMIN FUNCTION VERSUS PROTECTOR FUNCTION OR ROLE

A vitamin is an indispensable substance required in very small amounts to promote growth, or reproduction, or to maintain health or life. While adults need hundreds of grams of the energy nutrients—protein, fats, and carbohydrates—only a few hundred milligrams of all the vitamins together is enough. That's because only minute amounts of vitamins are needed to support the body processes we collectively call metabolism (the sum total of all the chemical reactions that go on in living cells). Indeed, in metabolism, vitamins are used over and over, and only small amounts are lost each time. However, since there are as many as twenty-five thousand reactions in some cells, the minute losses add up, so we need vitamins every day.

In contrast to their metabolic role, vitamins' protector capacity usually calls for them to be sacrificed in neutralizing lethal chemicals or radiation, such as ultraviolet light. Once a vitamin or any other protector is sacrificed in this role, it's gone. The byproducts of the interaction are eliminated and the protector must be replenished from food, body reserves, or supplements. Not all vitamins serve a protector function, and those that don't aren't discussed in this book.

RECOMMENDED DAILY ALLOWANCES, OR RDAs

RDAs are the amounts of nutrients that the Food and Nutrition Board of the National Academy of Sciences recommends we get from our food to maintain satisfactory health. Satisfactory health means freedom from symptoms of nutrient deficiencies for average, healthy people. RDAs usually have a large margin for error by this definition.

For example, only 10 milligrams of vitamin C daily will prevent scurvy, and 30 milligrams will maintain normal reserves that will keep you free from scurvy for a month or two if your vitamin C intake stops. By setting the RDA at 60 milligrams daily, the Food and Nutrition Board provides a generous excess to maintain reserves for about three months. However, in developing RDAs for vitamins, the protector role wasn't considered.

One in ten women get breast cancer, and a variety of risk factors have been identified for it. These factors include heredity and range through overweight, constipation, high-fat diet, and not enough vitamin C. That's right, vitamin C reduces the risk of breast cancer when you have vitamin C levels over six times the RDA. In these amounts, vitamin C isn't functioning as a vitamin; it's functioning as a protector.

RDAs are valid recommendations for people to maintain satisfactory health and be free from deficiency. In fact, the RDAs might even be excessive in that context. However, the protector role is not a vitamin function, so you've got to decide for yourself whether you want to have the levels required for this role. Prevention usually becomes an individual commitment. I think of it as a commitment to excellence in health.

Some of the protectors you'll learn about in this book aren't classified as required nutrients, let alone have the exalted status of vitamins. In fact, among professionals, some protectors aren't even thought of as nutrients. You might be more comfortable dealing with these substances, because there's no RDA dilemma to think about. All you need to do is weigh the evidence supporting them and decide whether or not you care. If you care for a longer, healthier life, I think you'll make a commitment.

ARE WE GAMBLING?

As you read this book, you will notice that I refer to risks and chances almost as though we're gambling. We all gamble with our health, even if we don't know it. Stand in front of an oncoming truck and you know what will happen. But if you start running to cross in front of the truck, I could bet on the outcome. My bet would depend on your starting point, your running ability, the speed of the truck, and other factors. Similarly, if you go into a room full of people with colds, I could bet on your chances of catching a cold. If you've just had a chill, have wet feet, had a poor night's sleep, and haven't been eating well, you have a high risk; I'd bet against you. In contrast, if you keep your health up, sleep well, avoid chills, wear rain gear in the rain, and take vitamin C, I'd bet with you.

When you hear scientists talk of "risk" and "odds," they're dealing in the same realm as someone who bets on horses. I use these words to explain what lifestyle steps you can take to reduce chances of getting a particular illness. It's a little like my example of entering a room filled with people who have colds. If health were an isolated, single event, we'd talk of odds and not risks, but since being healthy goes on every instant of every day, the odds are always changing; keeping healthy is an ongoing risk. And just as the risk of becoming ill is always present, your effort to reduce the risk should never take a rest.

Who decides risk? The odds at a horse race are decided by how people bet. If few bets are placed on a horse, it gets the longest odds, say 50 to 1. If everyone bets on it, the odds get closer to even money, or 2 to 1. In contrast to the odds at a horse race, some chances are certain; if you flip a coin, the odds of either heads or tails are equal or 50 percent. But on any five flips, you might get several heads in a row. If you pull a card from a standard deck, the chance of getting a diamond is one in four, or 25 percent. But on a few tries the result might be no diamonds or all diamonds.

In my three examples, the long-shot horse might win every race it runs for a month. As its winnings increase, the odds go down, because more people will bet on it. If you pull a card from a deck, you could get three hearts in three tries; but if you did it a hundred times, a heart would come up 25 percent of the time. The same with the coin flip; you might get three heads in three tries, but in one hundred tries it will be close to 50-percent heads. If the cards or the coin don't turn out the way we predict on one hundred tries, we look for a fixed deck or a weighted coin. Health risks are less certain than coin flips or card draws and move more like horse races. Health risks are determined by epidemiologists instead of by oddsmakers. Put in the converse, epidemiologists are the oddsmakers of life, and we are the bettors.

Epidemiologists study all the relationships in health and develop odds with respect to certain factors or aspects, so they can predict risks. For example, they have compared the rate of colon cancer in a group of people the same age and sex, with similar vital statistics, such as weight and height, and living in the same geographical location for several generations. They found that your risk of getting colon cancer increases as you eat more dietary fat and beef and if you're overweight, among other factors. They also found your risk declines if you eat the right amount and type of dietary fiber. Combining risk factors—say you eat a lot of beef and you eat no vegetables—means your risk is greater than if you just add together each factor. So having more than one factor complicates the entire risk picture.

In the research context, epidemiology is medical detective work, and epidemiologists are the detectives. They usually start with a disease or other health-related phenomenon and ask why one group of people has it or why they don't have it. Often the emphasis is on food or food-related habits. Epidemiology findings have been accelerated in the twentieth century through computer use, and epidemiology has led the way in health sciences research for the last three decades. Much of our knowledge about the protectors comes from epidemiological research, so you'll meet up with it throughout this book.

HEREDITY OR ENVIRONMENT?

Think back to my coin and card examples. If a coin always comes up heads, or if a deck always produces diamonds, it's fixed. In health we're always living with some factors fixed against us and some in our favor. We call it heredity. Look at it this way: Whom you chose for your parents is very important.

Just as our parents endow us with height, hair color, personality, and other factors we can see, they also pass on to us the tendency to get diseases. As scientists understand genetics better, we realize that every illness has an inherited tendency. Notice I said "tendency."

A tendency doesn't mean you'll get the disease. It simply means your risk is higher than average. A higher-than-average risk makes you more susceptible to environmental factors, such as a high-fat diet, or smoking. It also means you should be more aggressive with the positive actions you will learn about in this book.

Former president Jimmy Carter came from a colorful family. You could say that his family is the story of how America lives. His sister Gloria drove motorcycles. His mother served in the Peace Corps. His brother ran a general store. Jimmy graduated from Annapolis and became president of the United States. Jimmy Carter's two sisters, brother, and father died of pancreatic cancer before they were sixty years of age.

Are their tragic, premature deaths due to heredity or the environment? You can build a case for either cause, but heredity appears more likely, since they all died after the age of fifty. Since cancer usually takes about twenty years to develop, the Carter family cancer probably started sometime around the age of thirty, when they had already gone their separate ways.

If their cancer was initiated by something in their diet or to which they were exposed when they were children, you would have expected all of them to have it by now. On the other hand, if it was a hereditary predisposition, you could expect only one parent to get it and not all the children. The risk factors for pancreatic cancer—alcohol intake and smoking—favor heredity as the explanation.

Asian women get breast cancer at one-sixth the rate of North American women. While one in ten women gets it in the United States, one in sixty women gets it in Asia. Consequently, epidemiologists asked: Is the difference in these rates because of heredity or the environment? The answer wasn't difficult to find.

Asian women's daughters who are raised in North America have the same rate of breast cancer as American-born women. It's that simple; either our diet or our environment favors breast cancer no matter what your ethnic origins.

Ruling out environment completely is difficult, except that cities and water supplies in Asia would seem to have more hazards than in America. And since smoking seems to reduce the risk of breast cancer, you'd not expect other environmental issues, such as air quality, to be significant risk factors. Therefore, attention is focused on diet; ours either favors cancer or the Asian diet protects against it. In fact, it's a combination of both, with a dash of lifestyle thrown in.

THE CHALLENGE OF PREVENTION

The illnesses I'll discuss in this book are not "either/or" diseases. We can't say you'll get them or you won't. What we can say is that the protectors will reduce your risk of getting these illnesses, and while you might not prevent the disease completely, you can reduce it to a livable inconvenience. Medication can do the rest. Believe me, that's more than worth the modest effort required.

Illnesses to Prevent

Arthritis	Impotence
Bladder cancer	Inflammatory bowel disease
Bone brittleness	Kidney failure
Breast cancer	Kidney stones
Cataracts	Liver dysfunction
Cervical cancer	Lung cancer
Colorectal cancer	Memory loss
Emphysema	Migraine headache
Esophagus cancer	Periodontal disease
Gallstones	Premature aging of skin
Hemorrhoids	Scleroderma
High blood pressure	Skin cancer
Immunoincompetence	Visual insensitivity

Try to visualize what it's like to experience these diseases. I've quoted very briefly from people who actually have the disease or from relatives of those who died from the disease. These comments will give you a better idea of what you need to prevent.

• *Arthritis:* "I woke up one day and my ankles hurt—like someone had poured hot oil on them. I tried to stand up, but couldn't. They were all puffy and red. The doctor immediately said it was arthritis, but the tests weren't positive for almost a year. It hurts too much to kneel down in church any longer."

• *Bladder cancer:* "The pain got so intense that I couldn't talk. They removed my bladder, and the urine collects in a pouch. It's uncomfortable, but doesn't hurt like it did before the operation. I'm always scared the urine will spill out on the floor. I didn't go for the chemotherapy because they said the chances weren't very good anyhow, since it had spread through the bladder wall. I know I'm not going to live more than a year.''

• *Bone brittleness:* "What the doctors don't tell you is that they can't really repair these bones once they break. I'm scared to stand up, but they tell me I have to or it'll get worse. They make me use a walker.''

• *Breast cancer:* ''I'm still half asleep after the biopsy and the surgeon says he's scheduled me for a mastectomy. All I could do was scream; it was like a nightmare. Now, two years later, I don't mind not having my breast. I even got through the chemotherapy. But I know my missing a breast bothers my husband when we're in bed. Sure, the prosthesis makes me look fine in a dress, but I can't wear it to bed.''

• *Cataracts:* ''At first I thought the lights needed to be brighter. Then I thought I needed a new correction for my glasses. After the operation, when I could see again, I wondered why I had purchased so many bright, loud clothes. The doctor laughed and said that whenever a mature woman comes to him wearing loud colors, he knows it's cataracts. Your vision is reduced by the cloudy lenses in your eyes.''

• *Cervical cancer:* ''The nurse called and said my Pap smear was abnormal. She asked if I could come in for a follow-up examination, but I couldn't answer. I couldn't talk. The examination confirmed my worst fear. Since I've had our children, we agreed that the hysterectomy was best. But what they don't tell you is that you have to take hormones. The next fear comes when you read the pamphlet about the side effects of hormones. And then, you have to go through life wondering if they got it all.''

• *Colonic cancer (also called colorectal cancer):* ''Mom's cancer began as a sharp pain in the abdomen; then she noticed bloody stools. Surgery left her with a colostomy; then she had chemotherapy. It made me sick to watch her hair fall out. The doctors and nurses were always pleasant, with a forced, hollow pleasantness, but they never said anything more definite than they have patients still alive after ten years. Somehow I knew she'd die from it, but I never admitted I knew. We had to watch her waste away; she looked like an old lady on her thirty-fifth birthday. She seemed to resent us children after a while, because we would live and she wouldn't. When she finally died, it was a relief for all of us, especially Mom, but we never had the nerve to admit it; I've only told you.''

- *Emphysema:* "It's like I'm living out my worst nightmares, one of those where you're being chased but can't run. I go around with this oxygen bottle strapped to my wheelchair. The oxygen scares people, so they don't ask me over anymore."
- *Esophagus cancer:* "I'm alive; I thank God for that. But when I look in the mirror and see the scars, I just sit alone and cry."
- *Gallstones:* "I thought I was having a heart attack. It was almost funny when the doctor showed me how it cleared up if I would lie on my right side. By the time they operated, I was ready—death was starting to look like a pretty good alternative."
- *Hemorrhoids:* "It's like your rectum has something in it and you've got to go, but you know you don't. Sometimes they bleed and it's very uncomfortable sitting. They're like a bad headache in your rectum that won't go away, and there isn't anything the doctor can really do for it. She always says it'll run its course."
- *High blood pressure:* "It was just there. I wasn't sick; I was just told I had it. The medication didn't take my sex drive away and drives me nuts; I can't get an erection anymore. I know our lack of sex life bothers my wife, even if she claims she doesn't care."
- *Immunoincompetence:* "An infection to most people means taking some antibiotic for a week or so. To me it means I'll get arthritislike pains in my joints off and on for weeks. I'm afraid of the slightest scratch."
- *Impotence:* "The worst nightmare can't be this bad. I'm afraid to go out with women. I've been to so many doctors and had so many tests that I can guarantee they don't know what they're doing. The psychiatrists are the worst."
- *Inflammatory bowel disease:* "You're afraid to go anywhere for fear of an attack. People don't invite you out after a while because you have to excuse yourself so much. A luncheon is something you look forward to, but at the same time, you dread it. I'm afraid of the simplest shopping trip. No one understands."
- *Kidney failure:* "It's frightening. You hook up to this machine every two or three days and watch your blood pump through it. I feel great when I'm finished, but it only lasts for a few hours and then I'm depressed again. I think of suicide a lot."
- *Kidney stones:* "I can tell now when they're coming. It starts as a dull ache. I can't seem to get comfortable. Thank God they can destroy them with lithotripsy now. The pain can get so intense it can't be described."

• *Liver dysfunction:* "I didn't drink or smoke. The doctor said it was from a virus and the wrong foods. I'm always tired and sometimes people will come up and ask me if I'm all right. I guess it'll always be this way."

• *Lung cancer:* "I know I coughed a lot. I didn't think it would happen to me. I was always going to quit smoking soon. Now what should I do?"

• *Memory loss:* "I know I should know, but I can't get it out. They have a big word for it; too big to remember. I can't do simple arithmetic sometimes. The worst is when you get somewhere and don't know why you're there."

• *Migraine headache:* "It's not pain! Pain is when you drop something heavy on your foot; it hurts. This is like an evil monster in your head, constantly twisting. It doesn't stop hurting. You can't get used to it because the monster keeps twisting, so it stays intense."

• *Periodontal disease:* "My teeth are perfect and I never had to wear braces. My bad breath was something I always hated, but lived with. I've had the pockets cleaned; the next step is surgery. If someone had only told me I could have prevented this, I would have done anything."

• *Premature aging of skin:* "I was so pretty. How do you tell your kids you weren't always like this? It's easy for people to tell you to get an operation, but it's not their body or their money."

• *Scleroderma:* "It started as a rash. Then when I made snowballs, I noticed my fingers would turn white. Here I am thirty-eight-years-old and my skin is tight on my face. It looks translucent. There's no cure."

• *Skin cancer:* "I noticed a small dark spot on the side of my nose. I didn't go to the doctor until it looked pinkish and itched. Now I'm scheduled for surgery next Tuesday. I'm scared because the doctor said it can be more serious than many people believe. He said I should have come to him sooner."

• *Visual insensitivity:* "I couldn't see things. Oh, I could focus all right, but people would point to something and I wouldn't be able to see it. The doctor showed me how insensitive my eyes were by using lights. I'm thankful it could be cleared up in one eye."

WHO'S RESPONSIBLE FOR PREVENTION?

You're responsible! If we could reduce prevention to being inoculated, vaccinated, or even taking an aspirin a day, we could patent products and market them through the medical system, or give them as a public service. But prevention with food is different; it can't be patented or legislated into law.

If cabbage or asparagus helps you prevent cancer, it's still your decision to eat them. No one will do it for you. There will be no "big brother" to look over your shoulder and make sure you eat your deep-green to orange vegetables and fruit every day. It'll always be up to you, and that's better, because it puts you in control of your health and makes life more interesting and meaningful. I'll show you how to change old eating habits for new ones that will help you live longer and healthier.

PART

I

ANTIOXIDANTS

Oxygen is essential to life. We can go without oxygen for only a few minutes before brain damage begins. Oxygen's ability to combine with other elements, releasing energy in the process, is called oxidation. It's the basis of life and comfort. Besides supplying energy for our body, oxidation powers cars, homes, space ships, and just about everything else.

Some oxygen-using processes are unwanted; in a sense, toxic. These processes can destroy living cells in our body in the same way they cause cars to rust. We can paint our cars to protect them, but what can we do for the cells in our body?

Nature has been working for over ten billion years, and life has been on earth for four billion of those years. It would be surprising, indeed, if nature hadn't developed some protective substances to counteract unwanted oxidation reactions in our body. Scientists call these protector materials "antioxidants." Antioxidants live up to their name and block unwanted oxidative processes.

In her universal efficiency, nature asks protectors to wear more than one hat. In the following chapters, you'll read about some protectors that also serve as essential nutrients. Here we're concerned with them more as protectors than as nutrients. As protectors, they impose a new criterion of dietary need. To function as

15

protectors, we need about 50 percent more of these nutrients than is required of them as basic nutrients. Should our criteria for vitamin C's need shift from preventing known deficiencies to preventing cancer and cataracts? Similar issues are raised with the other protectors that are already recognized nutrients, such as vitamin E and selenium.

If a protector isn't recognized as a nutrient, such as lycopene, should it be given the status of a nutrient? Better still, should a new status be created for these protector materials? For argument's sake, why not call them protectors and let prevention be their criteria?

Think about these questions as you read the following chapters. If you notice yourself eating a few more or different vegetables or fruits, then take your actions as your answer.

As the antioxidant picture unfolds, you'll see how the antioxidant protectors work together. Indeed, they enhance the protection of each other—in protective harmony—proving that teamwork counts in nutrition.

1

Beta Carotene and Carotenoids

Beta carotene prevents sunburn and prevents cancer of the skin, lungs, mouth, esophagus, gastrointestinal tract, and bladder. Lycopene, the carotenoid that makes tomatoes red, prevents bladder cancer. Canthaxanthin, another carotenoid, prevents some cancers, especially of the skin. There are myriad carotenoids, and all of them help reduce the risk of cancer. That's enough to make me eat carrots, tomatoes, and green, red, and yellow vegetables regularly. If carotenoids prevent cancer, don't you wonder what they are, and what other diseases they prevent?

"Always have color on your plate" is an old wives' saying predating the Christian era. This bit of folk wisdom meant eating green, yellow, and red vegetables. Folk wisdom can be as good as modern science, because it has survived the test of time and evolved into traditions over many generations. This expression is the equivalent of a twentieth-century dietician saying, "Eat a wide variety of lots of vegetables." This advice is more important today than ever.

We know now that this advice insured that people would get enough carotenoids so their body could make vitamin A, with more left over to do what carotenoids do best—prevent cancer and even the effects of too much sun.

17

Carotenoid Quiz

Answer yes or no to these questions:

- Have you or any blood relative had cancer of the skin, mouth, throat, esophagus, tissues, lungs, or intestines?

- Do you work in the sun or spend recreational time in the sun with your skin exposed?

- Do you have light skin? blue eyes? Do you sunburn easily?

- Do you smoke or spend time with people who smoke?

- Do you chew tobacco?

- Do you work or live in a metropolitan area?

- Is your skin especially sensitive and normally dry?

If you answered yes to any of these questions, you should pay special attention to the carotenoids in your diet and the folk wisdom that tells you to "put color on your plate."

Carotenoids are pigments that impart color to plants and are important for plant growth and survival. Carrots are rich in beta carotene; red tomatoes and peppers are rich in lycopene. Yellow vegetables have a blend of several carotenoids and often contain canthaxanthin. At last count, there were five hundred and sixty-three known carotenoids classified into ten groups, and chemists expect to find even more as more plants are studied.

Beta carotene and other carotenoids are always associated with a specialized green pigment called chlorophyll. Both carotenoids and chlorophyll are found in a plant's leaves or other green tissues exposed to sunlight. As is not true for chlorophyll, carotene pigments are also found in roots, stems, flowers, and fruits and even in animal tissues.

Flamingoes, salmon, and lobsters eat plants that contain carotenoids. These pigments accumulate in flamingo feathers, salmon flesh, and lobster shells and give them their distinctive colors. If you eat lots of carrots every day for a month or so, you might notice the palms of your hands turning a little orange; it's beta carotene accumulation in your skin.

"Photo" means light and "synthesis" means putting together, so photosynthesis means putting things together with light. The chlorophyll in green plants uses energy from light to combine carbon dioxide from the air with water from the soil to make the simple sugar glucose and oxygen. All animals, including humans, use glucose and oxygen, then exhale carbon dioxide in their breath. This harmonic cycle of supply and demand involving photosynthesis is basic to all life on earth.

Chlorophyll traps only a very precise portion of sunlight to make glucose. Beta carotene also traps part of the sunlight, letting the right part of the light pass to the chlorophyll and so acting as a natural filter. Depending on the intensity of the light and the environment, including water vapor and gases, other carotenoids also block portions of sunlight and protect chlorophyll. But they do more than just filter light.

While light is a necessary energy source for chlorophyll, some parts of light create toxins called "free radicals" and "superoxides." Think of these toxins as submicroscopic explosives with quickly burning fuses. If they aren't put out or contained, they can do much harm. In living plant tissues, carotenoids neutralize these toxins. Carotenoids do the same thing in our body where these toxins are just as deadly.

Free radicals and superoxides are highly reactive materials that only survive for milliseconds; that's 0.001 of a second. They come in many forms; some are created when sunlight strikes normal, everyday chemicals, such as oxygen. Others are created in chemical reactions involving such commonly occurring chemicals as chlorine in water, carbon monoxide or nitrogen oxides in exhaust fumes, and countless others. We call some of these toxins superoxides because they contain an especially lethal and reactive form of oxygen. Free radicals have an electric structure that makes them especially reactive, too. Although they only survive for a tiny fraction of a second, they react so readily with everything that they take oxygen's place in the chemical reaction oxidation. The result is oxidative destruction. That's why I think of them as microscopic explosives that can destroy delicate biological structures, such as cell membranes or even nuclei.

All carotenoids have an abundance of internal structures that react easily with these superoxides, free radicals, and the toxins they produce. The carotenoids neutralize them, and they can be safely excreted from the body. So not only do carotenoids act as nature's sunblock, they also prevent noxious materials from destroying sensitive tissues.

When a free radical, superoxide, or ultraviolet light isn't neutralized, it, like an explosion, destroys some part of a living cell through oxidative destruction. If it destroys the cell membrane, the cell may leak vital material or let in toxins. If the nucleus of the cell is affected, the cell's genetic material may be changed, resulting in a precancerous cell. This neutralizing ability makes carotenoids part of a broad class of beneficial protectors we call antioxidants and free-radical scavengers. Stick with the explosion analogy, and carotenoids are some of nature's best bomb-defusing experts.

We believe now that all carotenoids evolved from beta carotene, since all five hundred and sixty-three carotenoids have the same central structure. Not surprisingly, beta carotene is the most widespread of all the carotenoids.

Plants use different carotenoids as they grow and mature. For example, two carotenoids abundant in tomatoes, lycopene and beta carotene, filter different parts of light. Beta carotene is the most effective carotenoid for protecting the tomato when it's green and still undergoing photosynthesis. Then, when the tomato ripens and photosynthesis is no longer occurring, lycopene takes over and protects the tomato against other toxins. The emergence of lycopene also announces that the tomato's ripe.

Different carotenoids work most effectively at different temperatures. Since the temperature changes inside the egg as it incubates, it's important to have protectors that function at the temperatures and conditions likely to be present. Egg yolks rely on beta carotene and canthaxanthin; beta carotene protects better at lower temperatures than canthaxanthin does. Both carotenoids come from chicken feed eaten by the egg-laying hen and give the yolk its color. An aside: canthaxanthin is sold in some countries as a "tanning" pill, because it colors the skin.

VITAMIN A

Over four thousand years ago in Egypt and Persia, people tested night vision with the third star, Mizar, in the dominant northern constellation, the Big Dipper. Mizar has a faint companion star,

Alcor, which means "a test" in Arabic. Alcor is just at the limit of vision, so if you could see it, your night vision passed; if not, it needed correcting. In Arabia, where this test originated and the star was named, people ate carrots or alfalfa to correct night vision.

By 450 B.C., Hippocrates, the Greek physician and father of modern medicine, used the same Arabic star-test to diagnose night blindness. But he had learned that it was more quickly cured by feeding the patient calves' liver than carrots. Calves' liver worked more quickly because it contains vitamin A, which was already made from beta carotene. When we eat beta carotene, our liver must first convert it to vitamin A before it can be used to improve vision. So, Hippocrates' cure was faster because he had removed a major step in the process.

Vitamin A is essential for the development of all tissue but is especially critical for eye tissue. Vitamin-A deficiency in under-developed countries accounts for at least sixty thousand cases of permanent childhood blindness annually. When there is not enough beta carotene or vitamin A in the diet of young children, eye tissues become keratinized. Keratinized tissue looks like a callous on your hand or foot, not clear, normal eye tissue. Obviously, you can't see out of a keratinized eye. This blindness can be prevented with a few cents' worth of beta carotene or vitamin A, but once keratinized tissue becomes established, it can't be reversed. Preventing blindness for the whole world annually would cost only a fraction of the cost of a single military aircraft.

What vitamin A does for your eye development, it does for all tissues throughout your life. These functions are all part of vitamin A's role as a vitamin; therefore, vitamin A is necessary for life. It's essential in all cell growth and development; it helps all body processes work by directing each cell to fill its intended role. For example, the cornea cells of your eye are clear and transparent, while a cell in your intestines is long and slender and produces mucus, yet they begin as the same kind of basic, undifferentiated cell. Vitamin A triggers the change. For example, our intestinal cells reproduce so rapidly that they're completely replaced about every three weeks. Vitamin A is absolutely essential for this process to occur correctly; similarly for all the fifty trillion cells in our body.

And, vitamin A is required for a good immune system that correctly identifies and kills foreign germs and cancer cells. In short, we can't live without vitamin A.

Of the five hundred and sixty-three carotenoids, beta carotene is the most efficient source of vitamin A. Some carotenoids are about 50-percent effective as sources for vitamin A and others aren't effective at all. For example, lycopene, which gives tomatoes their red color, is useless as a source of vitamin A. But lycopene serves as an antioxidant, tells us when tomatoes are ripe, and protects us from bladder cancer, so it earns its keep.

BETA CAROTENE

Beta carotene has emerged as a protector nutrient in its own right. However, before 1981, it was primarily considered nature's source of vitamin A. Vitamin A is essential for many bodily processes, but it's not a cancer protector or sunblock. To a chemist, vitamin A looks like one half of a beta carotene molecule.

In our body, mostly in the liver, beta carotene is broken in two, as needed, making vitamin A. I emphasize "as needed" because the body only converts enough beta carotene to satisfy its needs. Greatly excessive amounts of vitamin A are toxic, but beta carotene is very safe. That's why we say beta carotene is nature's preferred source for vitamin A. In fact, since the body stores beta carotene, you can look at it as a natural vitamin A reservoir.

Excess vitamin A is toxic. Vitamin A toxicity starts with loss of appetite and then progresses to development of a skin rash, kidney malfunction, and eventually death if the person continues taking high levels of vitamin A.

An adolescent boy requires 1,000 units of vitamin A daily; a somewhat smaller girl requires a bit less. Since 1,000 units of vitamin A are made from 6 milligrams of beta carotene, these requirements are met by 6 milligrams. A medium-size, 2-ounce carrot provides about 12 milligrams of beta carotene. If a carrot were the only daily source of beta carotene, the boy's body would use 6 milligrams for vitamin A and the other 6 milligrams would remain in his body as beta carotene until it was eliminated. While still in the body, beta carotene is a major protector.

SAFETY OF BETA CAROTENE

People with the skin disorders called porphyria, a sensitivity to light, require 300 milligrams of beta carotene daily. Three hundred milligrams would be fifty times the RDA if it were all converted to vitamin A. Over a period of weeks or months, fifty times the RDA of vitamin A would be toxic, but there have been no adverse side effects from the beta carotene and no vitamin-A toxicity from any of these therapeutic uses—proof that the body only converts the beta carotene it needs.

Children with porphyria have used 60 milligrams of beta carotene daily for years with no adverse side effects. A slight yellowing of the skin develops, which, for some people, is a side benefit, because it allows them to develop a nice tan. When beta carotene is used in such large amounts, it's being used as a drug. It's the only drug with a beneficial side effect (a tan) and no negative side effects. The important question is: Does the body need the extra beta carotene it gets from food?

Yes! Your body depends on beta carotene for other things besides fulfilling its need for vitamin A. We also believe your body depends on other carotenoids as well, although beta carotene is the best known.

In a 1968 paper, Norman Krinsky, a biochemist at Tufts Medical School, discussed how beta carotene protects us. Though scientists debate some details of Krinsky's hypothesis, they all seem to agree that beta carotene protects body cells from sunlight, free radicals, and oxidizing agents. I hope this sounds familiar, because Krinsky proposed that beta carotene does for us what it does for plants and a lot more. Though we don't photosynthesize, we are exposed to the sun and the same toxic chemicals as plants.

BETA CAROTENE AS A SUNSCREEN

Intuitively, wouldn't you expect that to happen? After all, we represent four billion years of development, and if something protects so well in plants, why wouldn't we use it for our survival?

Krinsky's hypothesis says that beta carotene finds its way into the membranes of all body cells. In cell membranes exposed to the light, it acts as a sunscreen. A sunscreen filters the harmful rays of sunlight from penetrating the skin. When these rays penetrate the skin faster than it can protect itself, the skin burns. Blood cells that get excessive sunlight can also be damaged.

Extra beta carotene is eliminated by becoming part of the cells of membrane tissues. Membrane tissues include the skin, the intestines, the lungs, and all other organs exposed to air. Skin, like all membranes, is reproduced about every six weeks from the bottom up. A short lesson in skin anatomy will help explain.

Skin consists of two major layers: the outer layer, or epidermis; and a lower layer, the dermis. The epidermis is made of two layers: an outer layer, the stratum corneum, consisting of dead, keratinized cells, and a basal layer of living cells. The basal cells reproduce and slowly move up to die, flatten out, and take their place in the stratum corneum, where they eventually slough off from washing, being rubbed by clothing, and by simply drying out. The dermis is a much thicker layer and contains nerves, blood cells, sweat glands, hair follicles, and many other small organs. Some organs, such as hair follicles, are actually appendages of the epidermis that extend into the dermis.

Practical experience tells you that beta carotene becomes a part of the dead skin cells of the epidermis, because if you eat enough carrots or take enough beta carotene, you'll become somewhat orange. The proof is that the orange color will come off, indicating that beta carotene is in these dead surface cells of the stratum corneum. Therefore, it follows that if beta carotene filters sunlight as Krinsky proposed, it works as a sunscreen: it filters the light that reaches the dermis.

All membranes reproduce in a similar manner—from the bottom up—and the outer, dead cells simply slough off. These cells also contain beta carotene and can develop a slight coloration, albeit not as intense as in skin. Obviously, you can't see the beta carotene that's in the cells that line your digestive tract, but they're there just the same, helping to protect these tissues from the toxins that we get from food and water.

The foundation for Krinsky's hypothesis appeared in an obscure report in 1926 in which people with skin disorders used lots of beta carotene to reduce their sensitivity to light. Then, in 1961, Dr. L. C. Harber, a physician at New York University of Medicine, treated a single patient who developed erythema from light. Erythema is a swelling, reddening, and rash on the skin. Dr. Harber gave the patient large amounts of beta carotene in capsules. Beta carotene delayed the onset of erythema when the patient was exposed to light, and Harber reported his results.

Dr. Micheline Mathews-Roth, a professor at Harvard Medical School, followed up on Harber's preliminary study. She began with animals in the 1970s and then selected people with severe porphyria. These people develop toxic chemicals under their skin when it's exposed to sunlight or even artificial light. These toxins cause swelling, fluid, itching, and reddening of the skin. It's a terrible illness that can be fatal if the sufferer isn't protected from light. Just imagine what life would be like if exposure to light caused such debilitating symptoms; you'd have to spend your life in the dark just to feel normal. What's worse, the disease is genetic and begins at birth; so children who have it will never be able to play in the sun or even bright light.

Dr. Mathews-Roth gave her patient-volunteers enough beta carotene to develop an orange-yellow discoloration of the skin. It took about four to six weeks to get this result, and the dose of beta carotene depended on the patient's age and size. One-year-olds got about 70 milligrams per day, while sixteen-year-olds got about 180 milligrams per day. Larger adult volunteers required as much as 300 milligrams per day.

The results were astounding: 84 percent of the patients could triple their exposure to sunlight with no symptoms. Life took on a new dimension, and these patients now engage in outdoor activities like anyone else. Some can even develop a suntan. Though you might not think of a suntan as an outstanding accomplishment for them, it's like allowing crippled people to not only walk unaided, but run as well.

Dr. Mathews-Roth proved that beta carotene is naturally transferred to the skin and modulates sunlight. An indirect outcome of the research is proof that, even if you take enough beta carotene to turn your skin yellow, it's safe. There weren't any toxic side effects from the beta carotene, but you could ask, What does this mean to me?

I'll let a blonde-haired, blue-eyed Viking Cruise Line hostess explain what it means to her. In her own words: "I get exposed off and on to a lot of sun. This intermittent exposure is the worst kind, because you can't control it. I rarely put sunscreen on as I don't particularly like to wear it when I'm in my uniform because it's so greasy; therefore, I decided to try beta carotene. I take 20 milligrams daily and have not had a sunburn since I started. Beta carotene is an excellent natural sunscreen for me.''

DOES BETA CAROTENE PREVENT CANCER?

Krinsky's hypothesis of 1968 also stated that since beta carotene neutralizes free radicals and superoxides, which arise after exposure to contaminants in the environment, it should prevent cancer of tissues exposed to the environment. This hypothesis simply applies beta carotene's normal antioxidant function in plants to people. It can't be said too often that these toxic oxidizing agents, including ultraviolet light, can cause problems, including cancer. Beta carotene blocks ultraviolet light and neutralizes many oxidizing agents.

The overwhelming evidence indicates that beta carotene does prevent cancer in tissues exposed to environmental carcinogens. It prevents skin cancer. It prevents cancer in the aerodigestive organs, including the mouth, throat, and esophagus. (The esophagus is the tube that connects your throat to your stomach.) Beta carotene prevents cancer of the lungs. Its action is most obvious in studies on heavy smokers, but it also works on passive smokers. (Passive smokers don't light up themselves, but there's so much smoke in the air they breathe, that we can think of them as light smokers.)

Beta carotene is moderately preventive for gastrointestinal cancers, including stomach, colon, and rectal cancers, commonly called colorectal. It prevents bladder cancer, and to a minor extent, breast cancer. Two studies have suggested it's even moderately protective for cervical cancer. Drug companies are searching for more effective carotenes for specific protection of high-risk people.

Table 1.1 summarizes the results of original studies on the prevention of human cancer by carotenoids, published in refereed medical journals between 1986 and 1990. I selected human studies because they get directly to the issues. Animal studies help biochemists understand what's going on, but at their conclusion, we all need to see the bottom line: Does it work in humans? And it's necessary to use refereed journals as sources of information. A refereed journal requires that all its published papers be reviewed by two or more experts in the same field as the authors. These experts make sure that the study meets the standards of scientific inquiry and that the investigators didn't reach unjustified conclusions—in other words, that they're based on results and not speculation. Using this standard meant I had to reject some papers in my analysis. This selection process left thirty-six studies to review. Thirty-four studies showed that beta carotene is clearly protective for one or more organs. One study was neutral for aerodigestive cancer prevention and one for digestive cancer prevention, but many other studies of these same organs showed positive protection. I concluded from this analysis that beta carotene is clearly protective against cancer.

Other scientific studies are presently being conducted to clarify the levels of beta carotene needed for protection and to identify the other carotenoids that are similarly protective.

TABLE 1.1

Beta Carotene's Protective Effect Against Cancer in Humans

Organs Protected	Summary of Published Findings
Lung	Strongly protective for active and passive smokers
Aerodigestive	Strongly protective in mouth, throat, and esophagus
Digestive (trends)	Protective in stomach, upper gastrointestinal, colon, and rectum
Bladder	Strongly protective; also strongly protective against a recurrence in people previously cured of bladder cancer
Skin	Protective against some but not all types of skin cancer
Breast (trends)	Somewhat protective but not a primary protector

On Table 1.1 I wrote "trends" by breast cancer and digestive cancer, because some studies didn't show a statistically significant reduction by the use of beta carotene, although the results were strongly tending in that direction. It really means that beta carotene seems to be protective in these tissues—though the study didn't include enough people to have a statistically significant result—or other protectors, such as fiber or vitamin C, were the dominant protectors. We're sure that more time and more extensive studies will more clearly show that beta carotene protects against these cancers, too, although other protectors may have a more dominant role.

Carotenoids protect us in two ways. The first way, antioxidation, is well understood. It may sound confusing, but I'll guide you through it in a moment. The other way, reversal of dysplasia (abnormal growth of organs, tissues, or cells), is right on the furthest edge of modern science. We don't understand it very well, at present, but when we do, I think cancer will become a disease of the past.

Antioxidation is like defusing a firecracker. We encounter many toxins that can destroy delicate biological membranes and even our genetic material by the chemical process we call oxidation. Think of oxidation as holding a lit firecracker in your hand that you can't simply toss away. The best thing is to snuff the firecracker fuse by cutting it off, throwing water on it, or by some other means. Well, that's one thing beta carotene does in our body. The superoxides and free radicals that are created in our bodies when we're exposed to carcinogens can cause the genetic material in normal cells to become abnormal: the nucleus or genetic control center of the cells becomes smaller than it should be. The result is cells that don't divide and reproduce properly. Beta carotene grabs the superoxides and free radicals and joins with them before they can disrupt oxidation.

Reversing dysplasia is like taking a child that's headed for a life of crime and getting that child to see the light and become a good citizen. Beta carotene does this at a level of genetic information. In this process, the cell is headed toward becoming cancerous, but it's not there yet. And like working with the erstwhile juvenile, beta carotene gets it to return to its normal path. This knowledge has become a major frontier of the science we call molecular biology.

BLOODY MARY

When I say that once you have cancer the protectors can't reverse it, I mean it. However, to be completely accurate, I have to admit there's a midstage where you don't actually have cancer, but you almost have it. It's called a dysplasia. A good example comes from Bloody Mary in the musical hit *South Pacific*.

You might recall that Bloody Mary chewed betel nuts, a habit that gave her lips and chin a blood-red color—hence the nickname "Bloody" Mary. Chewing betel nuts for a lifetime increases the chances of lip and mouth cancer. There's a stage when a good pathologist can look at cells from the mouth, lips, or throat and identify them as precancerous. These cells are micronucleated, which means the nucleus is not normal and they are displaced from normal toward becoming full-fledged cancer cells. A clump of them is a dysplasia and each one is dysplastic.

If a South Sea islander who chews betel nuts and has micronu-cleated cells stops chewing betel nuts and takes a lot of beta car-otene, most of the cells will eventually revert to normal. If he or she continues to chew betel nuts but also takes beta carotene, the likelihood of developing enough precancerous, micronucleated cells to get cancer decreases sharply. The lesson from this illustra-tion is simple and twofold: Don't chew betel nuts! If you chew betel nuts, take lots of beta carotene!

Another example of cancer prevention can be found a little closer to home among tobacco chewers, or "snuff dippers," as they're called. Tobacco chewing causes cancer by a process similar to betel-nut chewing and can be identified by the same method—finding a number of precancerous, micronucleated cells that are thus dysplastic. Many major-league baseball players chew tobacco. As a result, 16 percent of them have mouth sores that contain a high proportion of dysplastic cells. It's a time bomb for them.

In 1980, it seemed logical to give snuff dippers supplements of beta carotene and vitamin A. These two supplements produced a large reduction in micronucleated cells. At the time, the research-ers didn't know whether the reduction was caused by beta caro-tene, vitamin A, or the combination of both, so a follow-up study was designed to determine the answer. In this study, volunteers were divided into two groups: one group was given beta carotene and the other vitamin A. The results were definitive: Beta carotene worked alone; vitamin A didn't work at all. There's no doubt that beta carotene protects cells from irritants, such as chewing tobacco or betel nuts, that cause genetic damage to cells. The genetic damage causes these micronucleated cells to reproduce out of control and form a cancerous lesion. Some of these cancers can grow very rapidly; for example, some double in size every forty-eight hours.

OTHER CAROTENOIDS

Krinsky's hypothesis on the protective effects of beta carotene is really a carotenoid hypothesis. Since beta carotene is the longest recognized and most abundant carotenoid, it is the easiest carotenoid for scientists to collect solid statistics on. Some scientific studies were large enough to bring out the protective effect of other carotenoids.

Table 1.2 lists carotenoids that have emerged as effective protectors against cancer or other illnesses and the vegetables and fruits from which they are easily obtained.

TABLE 1.2

Protective Carotenoids

	Food Sources
Beta carotene	Mangos, papaya; dark green, orange, and yellow vegetables
Lycopene	Red fruits and vegetables, such as tomatoes and watermelons
Lutein	Dark green vegetables including broccoli, cabbage, lettuce, taro leaves, Swiss chard, spinach, bok choy, watercress
Canthaxanthin	Yellow vegetables and fruits; egg yolks

These carotenoids were proven effective before 1991.

Many epidemiological studies don't focus on only one carotenoid, but do identify certain vegetables and fruits as having protective properties. Since many carotenoids are abundant in these foods, they all are probably similarly protective, although much more research is required to determine the extent of their protection.

TOMATOES, ANYONE?

The bladder lining is an epithelial tissue exposed to concentrations of the same environmental toxins as aerodigestive tissues, lung tissue, and, to a lesser extent, skin and intestinal tissues. The risk of bladder cancer increases if you smoke, use snuff, or have been exposed to chlorinated drinking water and other environmental factors. Look at it this way: Most toxic materials you breathe or ingest with food are either eliminated directly in urine or indirectly as byproducts of the body's metabolism, so they're in prolonged contact with the bladder, giving them plenty of time to act on the epithelial tissue.

Many epidemiological studies examine the preventive nature of foods, not specific carotenes. Tomatoes showed up in several studies as being preventive. Then, by statistical analysis, this protective effect was narrowed down to lycopene, the red carotenoid pigment in tomatoes. This means that two carotenoids are protective against bladder cancer: beta carotene and lycopene.

Translated to food, this finding supports, even more, the folk wisdom of "color on your plate." Indeed, it suggests that tomatoes, tomato sauces, watermelon, and other red fruits and vegetables are important. A plate of spaghetti with tomato sauce and with watermelon for dessert is a protective powerhouse.

It's no accident that we search for illicit drugs, steroids, and other materials in the urine. The bladder is our body's toxic dump. Some of these materials are sufficiently toxic to cause bladder cancer; therefore, it's not surprising that the bladder cells are protected by carotenoids. The practical aspects can be expressed better by a conversation that took place on a TV talk show.

The TV guest was a research physician who had been instrumental in developing a screening test for bladder cancer. It's a test that is done like the pap smear test, which identifies dysplastic cells in the uterus, cervix, or vagina. The host allowed the physician to explain that and then got right to the heart of the matter:

The host asked, "Okay, doctor, suppose I take the test and it comes up positive. I'm scared to death, but what good does it do me to know? What can you do besides scare me?''

To which the doctor answered, ''I would immediately put you on beta carotene therapy.''

The ability of beta carotene to protect is clear, but this doctor's reply says more. Beta carotene can help dysplastic cells return to normal. Once a group of cells have become dysplastic, they're in a stage between normal and cancerous. The object of screening tests is to catch them while they're in this dysplastic phase and nurse them back to normal. That's what beta carotene seems to do.

Tomatoes are the most widely eaten vegetable in North America. Early Spanish explorers discovered them among the native food plants of South America. Once the explorers brought back the tomato seeds, tomatoes were cultivated in Europe and England as ornamental plants. The fruit, a berry, was avoided by some as the ''forbidden fruit'' of Genesis. Its use, however, was accelerated by others who saw tomatoes as the aphrodisiac that aroused Adam. Aphrodisiac users prevailed and tomatoes became known as ''love apples.'' By the 1600s, they were being used in salads, although their use was not widespread for another two hundred years.

One object of this book is to show you that vitamin-mineral content is not the only criteria for selecting food. Tomatoes rank about sixteenth by that criteria and are first in actual use, perhaps because their color makes them more attractive. Broccoli, in contrast, ranks number one in vitamin-mineral content and is number sixteen in actual use. By the criteria in this book, broccoli would probably still be number one, because it contains plenty of protectors. But if you've had bladder cancer, I recommend plenty of tomatoes.

More insight into the preventive power of carotenoids comes from studies on people who have already had bladder cancer. People who have been cured of bladder cancer have a high risk of getting it again. In view of this, scientists analyzed diets and carotenoid levels of people who have had bladder cancer, in their search for protectors.

People who have been cured of bladder cancer can reduce the risk of a second bout with cancer by 66 percent simply by increasing dietary carotenoids.

If you've been cured of bladder cancer, you're still in a high-risk group. If you eat a diet low in carotenoids, your chances of getting bladder cancer again are 1.8 times as great as someone who eats foods with lots of carotenoids. Analyzing risk ratios and statistics can cause confusion, but the bottom line is clear: carotenoids protect against bladder cancer, especially the second time around.

WHO NEEDS MORE CAROTENOIDS?

The amount of skin pigment we have is derived from how near the equator our ancestors developed. Some ultraviolet light from sunlight striking the skin penetrates to the blood below the skin and converts cholesterol to vitamin D. Since excess vitamin D is toxic, the skin darkens to reduce the amount of vitamin D produced. That's why people whose ancestors originated between the tropics of Cancer and Capricorn have dark skin. Other people native to areas close to that zone have a good ability to tan. People in the far north, such as those from Scotland or Lapland, have the fairest skin, lightest eyes, and light hair. Their skin is actually thinner and more transparent than the skin of people from further south. Living that far north, overexposure to sunlight wasn't a problem.

People with light skin, blue eyes, and light hair have a greater risk of skin cancer and cataracts. Both risks increase as they're exposed to sunlight and the products of industry. People endowed with these fair qualities have lower pigment levels to sunlight and similarly lower barriers to airborne toxicants. It follows that fair-skinned people should strive for more carotenes in their diet than people with darker skin or who have the ability to tan easily. Getting more carotenes can be accomplished by simply doing what the cruise ship hostess did: eat correctly and use beta-carotene supplements. Whenever I talk about how much of the carotenoids we need, people in the light-skin category should add about half again as much. It can't do any harm and packs a lot of preventive power.

EMPHYSEMA: SMOKE

People who expose their lungs to tobacco smoke and other irritants often develop emphysema even if they don't get lung cancer. Irritated and injured lung tissue develops scar tissue and loses its flexibility and ability to extract oxygen from the air. It's somewhat like the wrinkled, leathery skin some people get from spending a lot of their time in the sun. Having emphysema is like living in a bad dream where you can't breathe.

Anything that protects lung tissue from irritants that oxidize delicate cell membranes will slow the development of emphysema, just as it slows wrinkling of the skin. Beta carotene prevents lung cancer and emphysema.

Don't heave a sigh of relief and gloat if you aren't a smoker. Unless you live far out in the country and don't commute to a city, you're probably a "passive smoker." A passive smoker is a person who lives in an urban area or works where the air isn't clean. That's about 80 percent of us.

Smokers have carbon monoxide in their blood. The oxygen in carbon monoxide is more reactive than oxygen in the air, so it joins more readily with hemoglobin in red blood cells and doesn't release the hemoglobin as regular oxygen does, so less oxygen reaches your body's cells. Carbon dioxide is easily detected in the blood because it reduces the red blood cells' ability to extract oxygen. At a blood level of 2 percent carbon dioxide, your ability to extract oxygen from the air is measurably reduced. So is your vision, reaction time, and a few other physiological measures that relate to reduced oxygen-carrying capacity. This test doesn't count the effects of other chemicals in smoke ranging from nicotine to myriad things that could fill a chemist's lab bench.

One pack of cigarettes a day elevates the carbon dioxide level in your blood to 4 percent. Two packs a day can push it over 7 percent. Three packs a day is even higher, but it gets worse. Suppose you don't smoke but work or live in a large city, commute in traffic, or work around smoke and fumes. The carbon dioxide level in your blood will sometimes reach 4 percent and even push 6 percent. That puts you in a league with a pack-a-day smoker.

Suppose you live in an urban area where there's light industry, freeway or highway traffic, and you must go into a moderate-sized city or large town regularly. The carbon dioxide level in your blood will often exceed 2 percent. That ranks you with a half-pack-a-day smoker. You won't have the other chemicals in your blood, such as nicotine, but you still need protection, because carbon dioxide and other materials are excellent free-radical producers.

Anyone who smokes or lives in an environment with smoke or

fumes should strive to get lots of beta carotene. They should start a folk wisdom of their own, such as "Two carrots a day to keep the doctor away, and a sweet potato occasionally helps you smell the roses longer!"

HOW MUCH BETA CAROTENE?

No one knows for sure how much beta carotene we need. We only know that the average North American dietary intake, including Canada's, is less than 6 milligrams of beta carotene per day. Six milligrams daily isn't enough. Many experts say we should strive for a minimum of 15 milligrams of beta carotene daily. If you live and work in a city, use public transportation, are exposed to smoke and fumes, exercise heavily where you might be exposed to fumes, or expose your skin to the sun, you definitely need more carotenoids than someone living on an Iowa or Saskatchewan farm.

THE EXPERTS SPEAK

A paper by Doctors K. Fred Gey, Georg B. Brubacher, and Hannes B. Stahelin in the *Journal of Clinical Nutrition* dealt with the issue of how much beta carotene we need. It focused on blood levels of beta carotene and, by doing so, reached clear and unequivocal conclusions. If you're a nonsmoker, you should get at least 15 milligrams of beta carotene daily. The researchers didn't say how much beta carotene a smoker should get, but a safe bet would be a minimum of 30 milligrams daily; maybe more.

One good thing about the carotenoids is their safety. We know that they're safe even past the point where your skin turns orange. Taking that much beta carotene, about 60 milligrams daily for an average person, isn't necessary, but simply meeting the RDA for vitamin A, 6 milligrams daily, isn't enough either. Gey's recommendation of a 15-milligram minimum seems like good advice. That's only one and a half carrots a day.

RETINOL EQUIVALENTS AND CAROTENOIDS

A modern dilemma is that the Food and Nutrition Board recognizes the need for vitamin A but not for carotenoids. Consequently, the RDA expresses our need for vitamin A as retinol equivalents (RE). Beta carotene is converted to REs by our liver and intestines in a ratio that allows us to calculate 6 milligrams of beta carotene for every 1,000 REs. It doesn't tell us anything about the other carotenoids, such as lycopene.

Some carotenoids require 12 milligrams to make 1,000 REs, and other carotenoids don't convert at all. For example, lycopene from tomatoes isn't made into REs, but it prevents bladder cancer. Even though I can calculate beta-carotene equivalents in tomatoes, I can't tell you about the other carotenoids they contain. Therefore, you should use a little common sense. If a vegetable is red or deep green, it contains some carotenoids. Since beta carotene is more orange than red, we can conclude that if a vegetable is red, it might not contain as much beta carotene as other carotenoids. Let's look at a few examples.

TABLE 1.3

Beta Carotene Content of Some Common Vegetables

Vegetable	Color	Beta carotene Milligrams/ serving*	Other Carotenoids
Carrot	Orange	12.0	Some
Green cabbage	Green	1.3	Few
Red cabbage	Red	None	Many
Green pepper	Green	0.2	Few
Red pepper	Red	2.0	Some
Tomato	Red	1.0	Many
Spinach (raw)	Green	1.1	Few
Spinach (canned)	Green	5.0	Few
Sweet potato	Orange	16.8	Some

*½ cup

Table 1.3 contains a few examples of red and orange vegetables that contain differing amounts of REs or beta carotene, but common sense tells us they contain other carotenoids. Compare red cabbage to green cabbage. This list can help you decide what to eat. I included the example of raw and canned spinach; now you know what Popeye knew! Cooked vegetables give up their beta carotene more easily than raw vegetables do.

I know you've been taught that there are more vitamins in raw vegetables than cooked vegetables. That's correct for some, such as vitamin C and a few B vitamins that are destroyed by heat. But beta carotene isn't destroyed by cooking and is often locked into a fraction of the vegetable I call the "fiber matrix." This matrix is softened by cooking and beta carotene is more easily released. So while I encourage snacking on raw carrots and broccoli, they're also good for you cooked. An excellent source of beta carotene is sweet potatoes, which you don't ever eat raw.

SUPPLEMENTS

Improved technology has made beta carotene available in supplement form. Indeed, the studies of Mathews-Roth and Harvard Medical School all use beta-carotene supplements. If you choose to use a supplement, select one that provides at least 10 milligrams of beta carotene for daily use. When you add it to a reasonably good diet, you should get over 15 milligrams of beta carotene daily. Since we don't know how important other carotenoids are for protection, you can't substitute supplements for a good diet. Therefore, follow the same daily rules in food selection below even if you take a beta-carotene supplement.

In Table 1.4 I've summarized the best sources of carotenoids and listed the minimum level of carotenoids, because there are no data readily available that provide total carotenoids. Once the health value of the carotenoids is widely understood and recognized by the government, complete values will be developed. It will probably take about ten years.

TABLE 1.4

Good Sources of Carotenoids
(Each is expressed as a 1/2-cup serving)

	Beta carotene (milligrams)		Beta carotene (milligrams)
VEGETABLES			
Avocado	0.9	Spinach	5.0
Beet greens	2.2	Spring onions	1.5
Broccoli	0.9	Peppers (sweet red)	2.0
Cabbage	1.3	Pokeberry	4.3
Carrots	12.0	Pumpkin	16.0
Chard, Swiss	1.6	Seaweed (Nori)	3.1
Chickory	2.2	Squash (winter)	2.2
Collards	3.0	Squash (hubbard)	3.7
Dandelion greens	3.6	Swamp cabbage	1.9
Dock	2.1	Sweet potato	16.8
Kale	2.3	Red tomato	1.0
Lamb's-quarters	5.2	Tomato paste	2.0
Mustard greens	1.3	Turnip greens	3.1
Mustard spinach	4.4		
FRUITS			
Acerola	0.5	Mango	4.8
Apricots	1.7	Nectarine	0.6
Cantaloupe	3.1	Papaya	3.7
Cherries	0.6	Peaches	0.5
Loquats	1.0	Persimmon	2.2
Mandarin orange	0.6	Prunes (10 prunes)	1.0

You can see by inspecting table 1.4 that with a little effort, you can get 15 milligrams of carotenoids daily. It's as easy as these daily rules.

TO GET ENOUGH CAROTENES

- Eat a serving of red or orange vegetables every day; two servings is better; boiled or steamed vegetables are better than raw.

- Eat two green leafy vegetables every day.

- Eat a piece of fruit with colored flesh every day.

- Supplement when in doubt. Use 5 to 15 milligrams of beta carotene, depending on your diet.

Beta carotene is safe up to 60 milligrams a day.

2

Vitamin C

Humans, other primates, fruit bats, guinea pigs, and a few other animals can't make their own vitamin C. When their diet has no vitamin C, they develop scurvy, a deadly group of symptoms caused by vitamin-C deficiency. If vitamin C isn't added to their diet, they'll die. Scurvy was described before the fifth century B.C., but its cause and cure were first understood in 1747.

Beginning with Vasco da Gama's long voyage around the Cape of Good Hope in 1497, scurvy became the scourge of explorers. Over half of da Gama's crew were lost to scurvy. During the three hundred years of extensive exploration and naval warfare between the fifteenth and eighteenth centuries, more English sailors were lost to scurvy than the total in all naval battles England ever fought. In those times, a ship often carried twice its required crew to make up for those who died. So it's not surprising that in 1747, an English naval surgeon, James Lind, set out to find a cure for what was then a terrible and costly disease.

Lind used information taken from many sources, including Amerigo Vespucci's log of 1499, in which he named a Caribbean island Curaçao, meaning *cure* in Portuguese. Amerigo had left some scorbutic sailors to die on the island while he sailed south charting South America. On his return several months later, he found the sailors he had left for dead, alive and well. "Cure" seemed to him like a good name for the island.

Lind tested the Caribbean lime among other foods on sailors with scurvy. They improved immediately after eating limes and were cured in three weeks. Lind recommended the admiralty provide a half-lime daily with each sailor's rum ration, advice the admiralty took after fifty years. That's why English sailors became known as limeys.

Vitamin C Quiz

Answer yes or no to these questions:

- Do you eat processed meat, such as frankfurters, bologna, bacon, and so on?

- Have you or any blood relative ever had cataracts?

- Do you work in the sun or spend a lot of recreational time boating or skiing in the sun?

- Are you frequently under a lot of stress from work, your personal life, or a chronic illness?

- Do you work at a physically demanding occupation, such as carpentry, masonry, truck driving, police work?

- Are you a woman? If you are, have you or any blood relative ever had breast cancer?

A yes answer to any of these questions indicates that you should be concerned about the amount of vitamin C in your diet.

WHAT IS VITAMIN C?

Vitamin C is a water-soluble carbohydrate that's a close relative of two common sugars, glucose and galactose. Vitamin C is made in plants from glucose and is found in most parts of the plant, especially the fruit. So our major source of vitamin C is fruits and vegetables, although we also get vitamin C from cow's milk.

Most animals and fish make large amounts of vitamin C, so their raw flesh is a good source; however, cooking destroys vitamin C. When early missionaries went to convert the Eskimos, many got scurvy until they adopted the Eskimo habit of eating raw fish and meat.

VITAMIN C DISTRIBUTION IN YOUR BODY

Our body absorbs vitamin C better when bioflavonoids, a group of materials found in most plants and foods, especially citrus fruits, are present. Being water soluble, vitamin C is transported by the blood and found in every cell in the body. If the body has too much vitamin C, any excess is excreted harmlessly.

Most tissues, such as muscles, and organs, such as kidneys, are "passive" to vitamin C. In those tissues and organs the level of vitamin C is about the same as it is in the blood. When vitamin C in the blood is high, the level in the tissues is high and vice versa.

In contrast to the vitamin-C content of passive tissues, some tissues need a much higher concentration of vitamin C to function correctly. Tissues that require more vitamin C must expend energy to build these higher levels, levels much higher than are found in the blood. This process is like getting water from a well; it takes energy to pull the water up in a bucket or to run a pump. Your body works the same way.

If there's adequate vitamin C in the blood, the task is easier. Some tissues build vitamin C to one hundred times the blood level if you're eating a healthy diet with lots of vitamin C. If your diet is poor, your body has to work harder to reach the same vitamin-C level. Using the well comparison, it's as if the well is two hundred feet deep instead of twenty feet.

If the water in a well is too deep, even a good pump can't do the job. It's the same with your body. If blood levels of vitamin C fall below a certain threshold, the tissue levels drop proportionately. Though deficiency symptoms may not appear, these high-vitamin-C-need tissues can't function as they should. The high levels of vitamin C in these tissues and glands indicate that vitamin C is especially important to their function.

The adrenal and pituitary glands require vitamin-C levels fifty to one hundred times higher than in the blood. The central nervous system, eye lens, spleen, bone marrow, testes, leukocytes or white blood cells, and salivary glands have vitamin-C levels thirty to fifty times higher than in the blood.

Scurvy is a group of symptoms that represent the final stages of a longstanding deficiency. The first symptoms are probably mental or a minor infection and go unnoticed. It's not until the deficiency progresses to the point where a person appears lazy or shows a pallor that the disease is noticed. At that point, a serious decline in body function has been established.

Scurvy's symptoms progress in proportion to the decline of vitamin C in the tissues listed above. Although it was a mystery in 1747, we understand now why scurvy progresses in the order it does. Laziness comes from affected adrenal glands and poor metabolism from deficiency of the pituitary gland. Because these glands need the highest levels of vitamin C, a deficiency would affect them first, and it does. Then abnormal behavior when the central nervous system is affected, then infection when leukocytes do not have sufficient vitamin C, and eventually enough major systems break down and death occurs.

Common symptoms of scurvy that we read about, such as bleeding gums, teeth falling out, bruising easily, and swollen joints, follow the first symptoms—laziness and poor metabolism—and are what we call moribund symptoms. When they occur, death is not far behind. Death from scurvy is actually caused by heart failure because prolonged lack of vitamin C also causes the arteries to become clogged.

In most societies, scurvy doesn't exist anymore. It's prevented in average people by just 10 milligrams of vitamin C daily. Anyone who eats any fresh fruit, vegetables, and even rare meat, or drinks milk, will get the 10 milligrams of vitamin C that prevents scurvy. Scurvy became a problem among sailors, because vitamin-C requirements increase with activity levels, hot weather, exposure to sunlight, and stress. And sailors on long voyages before refrigeration had no fresh fruit or meat for months between landfalls. Scurvy is the exaggerated condition produced by a longstanding, very poor diet. The attention given to scurvy has actually taken attention away from vitamin C's critically important protector functions. Cancer prevention is the most obvious.

CANCER PREVENTION BY VITAMIN C

Both theoretical and experimental science meet at a common focus on the ability of vitamin C to prevent cancer. Theory leads researchers to expect vitamin C to block development of some cancer initiators. An initiator is something that can alter a healthy cell and cause it to be dysplastic. The cell then becomes cancerous under some conditions, such as the presence of excessive fat, that promote cancer. The theory can be tested experimentally by the biochemist; then the epidemiologist can study people to see if dietary practice supports theory and experiment. Vitamin C emerges from this research as an important protector.

Ask a group of people if nitrates cause cancer, and they'll usually say yes. They're wrong. Nitrates don't cause cancer, but a very close relative, nitrosamines, do. The reason we focus on nitrates and nitrites is that they are converted to nitrosamines in food and in our body. So, indirectly, nitrates cause cancer, but they won't if they aren't first converted to nitrosamines. That's where vitamin C comes in.

Nitrates and nitrites are found naturally in green vegetables, such as spinach, broccoli, and lettuce, to name a few, and are added to many processed meats, such as hot dogs, bacon, smoked meats, and luncheon meats. Nitrates are also found in most municipal drinking water, water from wells, and even bottled water. Nitrates and nitrites are converted to nitrosamines in our body. Nitrosamines cause cancer.

Scientists estimate that, on average, we get at least 75 milligrams of nitrates and probably more than 150 milligrams of nitrites and nitrates daily from food and water consumption. Under many conditions, such as a diet rich in processed meat, we may get much more. This nitrate problem has been verified by research in the United States, United Kingdom, Canada, Italy, China, and other countries. Wherever nitrates are widely used, cancer rates are higher.

Since 1969, we've known that vitamin C reduces the building of nitrosamines from nitrates. In 1975, Dr. John Weisburger of the American Health Foundation proved that having a 4 to 1 ratio of vitamin C to nitrates present prevented over 97 percent of expected nitrosamine formation! Increase the ratio and you'll get 100-percent protection.

Weisburger did an experiment in animals that has far-reaching implications in human cancer. He gave nitrated fish to rats and added vitamin C to some of the nitrated fish. Then he put the rats on an anticancer diet, the rat equivalent of the Longevity Diet in chapter 15. Rats that ate the nitrated fish without vitamin C got cancer in spite of the protective diet after exposure. Rats that ate nitrated fish with vitamin C—thus getting the vitamin C at the same time as the nitrate—didn't get cancer.

John Weisburger's experiment confirms that exposure to nitrosamines initiates cancer; but it also implies that prevention of nitrosamine formation prevents cancer. Waiting until after the exposure to nitrates to get vitamin C is like closing the barn door after the horse has escaped. Although it would be unethical to repeat these experiments in humans, epidemiologists have confirmed their conclusions by showing excellent correlations between nitrate exposure and cancer.

We'll see that these studies and others like them raise serious concerns about our daily need for vitamin C. Think about this question as you read on: Should the daily need for vitamin C be based on research principles derived from avoiding scurvy, or should it also consider the nitrate level in our diet?

WHAT'S A FREE RADICAL?

We're not talking about the radical who goes around with a knapsack and a sign, or a young man with a beard who comes from Berkeley, California. The free radicals we talk about in prevention are at a level you can't even see with an electron microscope and are so reactive that they last for less than one millisecond (one one-thousandth of a second). In precise terms, that's 0.001 second or less!

I like to think of free radicals as powerful, biological firecrackers. Remember when I said to think of beta carotene as defusing a lit firecracker? Now think of the firecracker as a free radical that causes the destruction of delicate, biological membranes. These membranes are even more delicate and microscopically smaller than the membranes in your mouth or the surface of your eye. They are at or below the level of the cell. If you want to be technical, use terms like *fine structure* and *ultra structure*. They're small.

So think of free radicals as biological firecrackers; and, like firecrackers, they come in all sizes, shapes, and forms. In fire-crackers, there's the little one-incher lady crackers, golf-ball-sized "cherry bombs," and so on. Some firecrackers you light and others you throw. Biological firecrackers also come with many names.

Free radicals have one thing in common: they oxidize the delicate biological materials in membranes. You'll read about and hear terms like *superoxides, peroxides, oxidizing agents,* and most often, *free radical.* I'll try to stick with *free radical* in this book.

All free radicals develop within our body as a result of chemical reactions or from radiation. The most common form of radiation is ultraviolet light. However, there's always some background radiation from the cosmic rays that permeate our universe. We can protect ourselves from ultraviolet light with sunscreens and sunglasses, but we can't avoid cosmic rays. It's another reason the protectors play such a significant role.

Most important, when the free radical reacts with a biological membrane, that membrane is forever changed. If a cell membrane is changed, the membrane can no longer function normally to keep out dangerous substances, and the cell becomes open to attack by other toxins. If the attack occurs at a finer level, say in the nucleus of the cell, it might change the genetic material. Once the genetic material has been changed, the cell is dysplastic. And a dysplastic cell can lead directly to cancer.

A DEMOLITION EXPERT: FREE-RADICAL BLOCKING

Vitamin C directly blocks some free radicals, such as components of smoke and fumes from solvents. However, its most important role could be its two indirect effects on other free-radical blockers.

Vitamin C restores an important free-radical blocker called glutathione. When glutathione stops a free radical or is used in metabolism, it is put in an inactive form, but vitamin C restores it to power. Vitamin C is rendered inactive in the restorative process, but it's easily replaced by diet. Glutathione, a natural protector that our body makes itself, depends on another protector, selenium. It's involved in many biochemical processes in all body tissues.

Vitamin C also enhances the protective role of vitamin E. Vitamin E is the collected activity of about eight materials, of which one, alpha tocopherol, dominates. (They will be discussed in chapter 3.) Vitamin C enhances vitamin-E activity by reducing the need for its use in processes that vitamin C can handle alone. Thus, the amount of vitamin E that would have been called for in these processes is used in other reactions. If you're deficient in vitamin C, the vitamin E in your body is called upon to do more work—its own work and the joint vitamin-C reactions. A simple example helps make this clearer.

Vitamin E protects lung tissues from nitrogen dioxide toxicity. Nitrogen dioxide is a common component of automobile fumes. However, if you're short of vitamin C, you'll be more susceptible to nitrogen dioxide toxicity, because your vitamin-E activity drops by about 25 percent to cover for vitamin C. So even though you may get plenty of dietary vitamin E, inadequate levels of vitamin C force reduction in its availability. This cooperation between the vitamins illustrates what I believe is twentieth-century folk wisdom: "In nutrition, teamwork is important."

RESISTANCE

When a rat develops a tumor, is assaulted by an infectious agent or toxic chemical, or is placed under stress, its body produces much larger amounts of vitamin C and its blood levels will increase much above normal. From these observations we conclude that vitamin C is essential to fight any serious stress. Therefore, when an animal that can make vitamin C is attacked, it responds by increasing its blood levels of vitamin C to meet the increased demands for vitamin C. This happens in any animal that makes vitamin C.

When your body is similarly attacked or placed under stress, its vitamin-C level drops because your body is using more vitamin C to counter the attack, but you don't make vitamin C. An important change is the drop of vitamin-C level in leukocytes, the white blood cells, when you're under physical or emotional stress. This drop in vitamin C explains why a chill (physical stress) often brings on a cold. You get a chill, which stresses your whole body, so your vitamin-C level drops throughout your body. Leukocytes are the first line of defense. When the leukocytes and other immune materials called antibodies drop below normal because of inadequate vitamin C, cold viruses can multiply. Vitamin C speeds the production of immune materials, which is why vitamin C makes the cold less severe. In vitamin-C deficiency, the number of these cells drops as much as 25 percent, and those that survive lose as much as 25 percent of their ability to attack foreign agents. It adds up to a 50-percent loss.

Armed with the change in rats, medical researchers studied levels of vitamin C in the white blood cells of cancer patients. They were low, in some cases at the level you'd find in scurvy. Then they studied people who had undergone surgery. Their vitamin-C levels, too, were as low as those you'd see in scurvy. Indeed, in the 1960s, some surgery patients were found to actually develop symptoms of scurvy in the hospital. A hospitalized person usually eats poorly, and the highly processed food is often overcooked. Overcooking destroys vitamin C, and eating poorly means you don't get the little vitamin C that's there.

So while rats can make vitamin C to compensate for the natural vitamin-C drop produced by severe stress, humans can't. We have just one recourse: eat more vitamin-C-rich foods or take supplements. Under some forms of stress, such as physical injury and even surgery, this isn't possible. White blood cells also attack and devour some cancer cells, so this has even broader implications.

DOES VITAMIN C PREVENT CANCER?

Theory, biochemistry, and epidemiology all point in the same direction: vitamin C protects against some types of cancer. In fact, theory, biochemical research, and practice meet at a common focus in cancer prevention.

Most epidemiological studies must sort through enormous amounts of dietary information. These studies are very good at separating macronutrients, such as fat, carbohydrate, and fiber, or specific foods, such as garlic or cabbage. However, they usually aren't sensitive enough to detect the different responses from micronutrients, such as vitamin C, unless there's a powerful effect.

When medical detectives seek to find a change in cancer risk related to vitamin C, they look at organs and tissues where there's most likely to be an effect. You would expect to see a positive effect from vitamin C in the aerodigestive tissues, such as the mouth and throat, which are exposed to nitrates that are bathed by saliva containing vitamin C. So these tissues are exposed to the risk agent—nitrates—as well as the possible preventor—vitamin C.

These tissues are especially susceptible to and exposed to such risk factors as smoking. These factors also reduce the circulating levels of vitamin C, making the saliva less protective. Alternatively, you would expect small effects in tissues such as the bladder, because they are exposed to different types of toxins. In fact, cancer protection in the bladder is led by lycopene and other carotenoids.

Results from the extensive epidemiology studies are summarized in Table 2.1. The number of cases of human cancer and people evaluated in these studies totaled over 46,828, and some studies followed people for over eleven years. This table summarizes the many studies and supports an unequivocal conclusion: vitamin C protects us against cancer!

TABLE 2.1

Vitamin C Protection Against Cancer

Tissue or Organ	Degree of Protection
Aerodigestive Larynx Mouth Esophagus	Strong protection (this cancer is related to nitrates and other toxins)
Stomach	Mild protection
Pancreas	Strong protection (the cancer is probably from digestive factors and resistance)
Colon and Rectum	Mildly protective; not as effective as fiber and carotenoids. Vitamin C helps to reduce polyp growth. Teamwork with fiber and carotenoids is important.
Lung	Slightly protective; works with vitamin E
Breast	380 milligrams or more of vitamin C daily reduces risk by: 16 percent in premenopausal women; 24 percent in postmenopausal women
Cervix	Strong protection above 30 milligrams daily

| *Childhood brain tumors* | Strongly protective if the mother got adequate vitamin C during pregnancy |
| *General cancer* | Mildly protective of most sites |

Table 2.1 rings out a clear message: our dependence on the protection that vitamin C can give us shouldn't be underestimated. Even more importantly, results from studies of childhood brain tumors suggest that protection begins in the womb.

When the results on childhood brain tumors came in, scientists at first didn't believe them. Epidemiologists examined and reexamined the results from many different points of view. The bottom line is clear: pregnant women who don't get adequate vitamin C have children who are more susceptible to brain cancer in childhood. The epidemiological findings bring to mind the old saying: "As the twig is bent, so grows the tree."

VITAMIN C PREVENTS BREAST CANCER

One out of ten women in the United States will get breast cancer. Therefore, in 1989, just over sixteen women were diagnosed with breast cancer every hour in the United States and Puerto Rico. If detected early, breast cancer is almost never fatal. However, since people usually put things off—and that includes doing self-examination as well as going to the doctor—43,200 women actually died from breast cancer in 1989. That's five women every hour.

In 1990, *The Journal of the National Cancer Institute* carried a paper summarizing many epidemiological studies. The significance of the report is clear: 380 milligrams of vitamin C daily from fruits and vegetables reduces the risk of breast cancer by 16 percent in premenopausal women and by 24 percent in postmenopausal women. That's a 20-percent reduction, on average. Let's apply the impact of that finding to the rate of breast cancer.

Instead of over sixteen women per hour diagnosed with breast cancer, the number would fall to thirteen. Instead of five dying every hour, four would die. The studies factored out the effects of beta carotene, fiber, and exercise, so the protectors are reduced to vitamin C; about four cents' worth daily. If you apply these other protectors, you can reduce your risks even more.

Most of us have read articles or heard dieticians and doctors say it's a waste of money to take supplemental vitamin C because everyone gets enough from diet and your body just excretes the excess. Yet this research, paid for by our tax dollars, says there is a 20-percent internal rate of return for any woman on the purchase of some extra oranges or a 500-milligram vitamin C tablet daily. If I told you that I could give you a 20-percent return on an investment, you'd jump for it. So why not do the same for your health?

So why do so many women ignore this preventive opportunity and so many people say taking vitamin C is a waste of money? Is it a waste of money to spend about sixty-cents per person daily on soft drinks? Or about one dollar per day for a woman to make her hair nice? How does it stack up against the one dollar daily per person spent on alcoholic beverages? How would these people compare it to the over one dollar we spend daily per person on cigarettes? Whenever someone says supplements are a waste of money, ask: "Compared to what?" This is an issue our policymakers must resolve.

The Longevity Diet provides about 100 milligrams of vitamin C, on average. So these important findings dictate that you should either eat three extra servings of a vitamin-C-rich food or take a tablet containing 250 milligrams or more of vitamin C. It's cheaper to take the supplement and no extra calories need to be fit into your diet.

Cancer is an oppressive topic, but there are also other illnesses to avoid that detract from an abundant life. Let's look at these illnesses and get a feeling for the other aspects of vitamin-C protection.

CATARACTS

Vitamin C is concentrated in the eye lens at a level thirty to fifty times greater than that found in the blood that surrounds the eye. What purpose does vitamin C serve there? A group of Australian researchers did a simple experiment. They gave one group of people extra vitamin C and vitamin E for five years and gave another group a placebo—an inactive substance used in controlled experiments testing the efficacy of another substance, such as a drug. The placebo group had 80 percent more cataracts than the group that received extra vitamin C and E. These results have been confirmed in other studies and different countries. Vitamin C protects us against cataracts. It works with vitamin E in this protective role. Teamwork!

SPERM AGGLUTINATION

Testicles contain at least fifty times more vitamin C than the blood that nourishes them. This observation prompted a group of physicians at the University of Texas Medical School to do an experiment on men who were infertile due to sperm clumping. Scientifically it's called *sperm agglutination.* These men were divided into two groups. One group was given a supplement of 500 milligrams of vitamin C daily and the other a placebo. The researchers then monitored the motility and clumping of the sperm produced by each group. Men who received the 500-milligram vitamin C supplements produced normal sperm and became fertile. Those who received the placebos remained infertile.

All male infertility is not the result of marginal vitamin-C deficiency or sperm agglutination. However, only these men had low, dietary levels of vitamin C. These studies confirm that the high concentration of vitamin C in the testicles serves an important reproductive purpose. More, this study suggests that some men may require more vitamin C than others.

BLEEDING GUMS

Who hasn't had bleeding gums from time to time? Some people always seem to have bleeding gums. This condition is called *gingivitis.* Gingivitis is one indication of poor periodontal health and leads to most tooth loss. The bleeding is associated with the growth of bacteria between the teeth and gums. Although bleeding gums are a symptom of scurvy and therefore of vitamin-C deficiency, lack of adequate vitamin C was not suspected as a cause of gingivitis because gingivitis has an identified bacterial agent and because scurvy is almost never seen in the industrialized countries. But Robert Jacobs at Tufts Medical School developed the hypothesis that people with this problem required more vitamin C.

People with bleeding gums were given a 600-milligram supplement of vitamin C daily. After several weeks the bleeding subsided and the condition of the gum-tooth interface improved. It's important to recognize that 600 milligrams is ten times the RDA for vitamin C. Research is continuing to find the minimum level required for protection. It's expected to be about 300 milligrams. This research doesn't mean that all bleeding gums are caused by inadequate vitamin C, but it proves that some people who get bleeding gums require more vitamin C than others.

In average people, the body's basic pool of vitamin C can be maintained by about 60 milligrams of vitamin C daily, the RDA. However, the body's basic reserve of vitamin C doesn't become full to overflowing until we get 100 milligrams daily, on average. Also, 100 milligrams isn't the 320 milligrams that reduces the risk of breast cancer by 20 percent. I'll explain what this means by comparing the body's reserve to a water reservoir.

Let's say a reservoir can supply enough water if there's sixty inches of rain each year. At sixty inches, the reservoir usually appears about three-fourths full, and no water flows over the dam. If there's a one-year drought, people can conserve water, and things are okay. Two years of drought, and things get bad. Severe rationing becomes necessary.

Things are better if the reservoir is completely full, say right to the top of the dam. With water to the top of the dam, the community can handle an extra year of drought; in fact, it could hold on for five years in a prolonged drought by very tight rationing.

In either example I didn't say what happens if there's a series of devastating fires, a serious water leak develops, or a customer, such as a factory, starts using an unusually high amount of water before someone finds out. Any of these things calls for a better, ongoing supply.

The best situation occurs when rainfall on our hypothetical village is about 100 inches per year. Streams keep feeding the reservoir, so it's 100 percent full, and a modest amount of water always flows over the dam, even in the summer. When this level of water prevails, the community is in its best position. It's ready for any emergency, such as fire, leaks, or extra demand. Not only can it handle demand, it can take a longer drought, because streams will continue to feed after the drought starts until they actually dry up themselves; and the dam can be closed to build a little over the average 100-percent level.

Our body works in a similar way with vitamin C. At 30 milligrams daily of vitamin C there are no symptoms of scurvy, and you could go about a month without additional vitamin C. However, you couldn't handle any serious illness or stress, nor would this level of vitamin C compensate for nitrates in your diet. Like the low reservoir, if nothing serious happens, you'd get along just fine.

At 60 milligrams daily of vitamin C, your basic vitamin-C reservoir is at the three-fourths level. You can handle stress, and your organs with a high requirement for vitamin C can build up the levels they require to function satisfactorily. Nonetheless, most scientists don't believe the 60-milligram level will give good protection from cataracts, and it's only one-sixth the amount required in the breast cancer studies. We do know that no symptoms of scurvy would show up for about ninety days even if you stopped taking vitamin C.

At about 100 milligrams of vitamin C daily, the basic body pool is full, and a small amount flows over our dam. That means that at 100 milligrams daily, average people will have some vitamin C in their urine. But don't get the notion that 100 milligrams will be enough, because there's a lot we still don't know.

John Weisburger created serious concern when he showed that a vitamin C to nitrates ratio of 4 to 1 prevented nitrosamine formation. If we get 150 milligrams of nitrates daily, the ratio says it would take six hundred milligrams of vitamin C to prevent the conversion of those nitrates to nitrosamines. However, let's take a closer look at sources of nitrates.

Vegetables such as spinach and broccoli that contain nitrates also contain vitamin C. So if they aren't cooked excessively, the nitrates they contain are probably blocked by the vitamin C they contain. But nitrate levels in vegetables vary more than vitamin-C levels. For example, spinach harvested on a cloudy day will contain more nitrates than that picked on a sunny day. The nitrate level also depends upon soil conditions. So in some cases, the spinach has enough vitamin C, and in other cases it doesn't.

What about nitrates that occur in drinking water or processed meats, such as hot dogs, bologna, and bacon? They aren't fortified with vitamin C, and there are other toxic agents besides nitrates, so there's no clear answer. It's important to recognize that we each consume about eighty hot dogs annually. That's a lot of nitrates. What about all the luncheon meats and smoked meats?

Nitrates have another sneaky feature: fat aids their conversion to nitrosamines. So not only do processed meats contain nitrates, their composition, with over 50 percent of their calories as fat, favors nitrosamine production. This issue of nitrates is avoided by policymakers when discussing our need for vitamin C because nitrates are so variable and policymakers must be concerned with basic satisfactory health. In our reservoir analogy, that's the three-fourths-full reservoir. Some countries go for the 30-milligram reservoir and others take the 100-milligram reservoir. None of them tend to give consideration to nitrates, cancer, cataracts, bleeding gums, clumping sperm, or respiratory problems, so we're going to deal with these issues here.

Another concern for vitamin C is stress. In my reservoir analogy, this is the catastrophic fire that can't be foreseen; it just happens. Suppose you get sick, are exposed to a cold, flu, or other illness. Do you need more vitamin C? Exposure to smoke, increased physical activity, prescription and nonprescription drug use, and aging all increase our need for vitamin C.

TABLE 2.2

How Much Vitamin C Is Necessary?

Purpose	Amount Needed Daily, in milligrams
BASICS	
To prevent scurvy (modest reserve)	30
To maintain full reserves	100
To combat smoking or bad air	150
IMPOSED EXTRA NEEDS	
To neutralize nitrates and other toxins	300 to 600
To combat stress	100
Individuality (gum problems, etc., see text)	Up to 500
To counter heat, sun, etc. (prevent cataracts)	Up to 500
For increased activity (athletes, laborers, etc.)	Up to 500
To reduce cancer risk	At least 380
To balance aging (by age 60)	50 percent more

I've divided table 2.2 into two parts so we can deal with each level of need directly. Basic needs of 100 milligrams will be met by the Longevity Diet with some left over for the second level of needs imposed by our lifestyle, toxins in the environment, and other factors. Inspect table 2.2 and then answer some questions:

- Do you smoke? If yes, add 150 milligrams of vitamin C.

- Do you eat processed meats? If yes, add 500 milligrams of vitamin C.

- Do you live with above-average, heavy, emotional or physical stress? Be honest. If the answer is yes, add 100 milligrams of vitamin C.

- Do you work outside in the hot sun? If yes, add 500 milligrams of vitamin C.

- Does cancer run in your family? If yes, add 500 milligrams of vitamin C.

Now add up the extra vitamin C. Depending on your work, lifestyle, habits, and heredity, you could justify taking an extra 500 to 1,500 milligrams of vitamin C daily. That should be more than enough vitamin C for most people. However, if cancer runs in your family or you work outside in the hot sun, taking more vitamin C couldn't hurt.

Surprisingly, many experts would differ with this advice. They might say you don't need it; you're wasting your money. Still other experts, including some Nobel Prize winners, would say 1,500 milligrams is too little. You've got to decide for yourself, but remember that more vitamin C won't do any harm and the overwhelming evidence suggests it'll do a lot of good.

NATURAL SOURCES OF VITAMIN C ARE IMPORTANT

Epidemiology focuses on vitamin C through foods and extensive dietary analyses. This research can factor out other recognized nutrients, such as the carotenoids, but it doesn't deal with dietary factors, such as bioflavonoids, associated with vitamin C. These food components may either enhance the action of vitamin C or substitute for it completely. A historical perspective will help you see what I mean.

BIOFLAVONOIDS

Although I hope this chapter will get you to take extra vitamin C every day, I don't want you to avoid natural fruits and vegetables because natural foods contain factors we call bioflavonoids. Until the 1980s, bioflavonoids were only thought of in connection with health food faddists. However, by examining one particular historical event, one scientist proved at least some of them are very important.

A LESSON IN HISTORY

In 1534, when Jacques Cartier and his men explored what is now Quebec, Canada, the frozen St. Lawrence Waterway forced them to spend the winter in their boats. Subsisting on salted meat and biscuits, the sailors soon began showing signs of scurvy. Scurvy could have brought disaster to the expedition, but the men were saved by a tea brewed by local Indians.

For four hundred and fifty years, scientists assumed this tea brewed from the bark and needles of pine trees contained vitamin C. Dr. Jack Masquelier at the University of Bordeaux proved the tea contained no vitamin C but contained a bioflavonoid. All plants contain bioflavonoids. Over five hundred bioflavonoids have been identified. Some of them can substitute for both vitamins C and E; some can substitute for one or the other.

Virtually all five hundred bioflavonoids have some antioxidant properties. It was probably the bioflavonoid pycnogenol in the needles and bark of the pine trees that saved Cartier and his men. Pycnogenol is fifty times better as an antioxidant than vitamin E and twenty times better than vitamin C. In contrast to vitamin C, it can withstand high temperatures, so it would survive the tea-brewing process.

This lesson is significant, because it emphasizes that while vitamins C and E are important, so is food. Just as there are myriad carotenoids that protect us from toxins, there are many bioflavonoids that protect us as well. Although we usually focus our attention on single vitamins, we should recognize that food contains many other materials that scientists are still studying and learning about every day. And some of them, like pycnogenol, have important protective properties.

SAFETY OF VITAMIN C

Linus Pauling started a vitamin-C revolution when he and his followers advocated that people routinely take from five to as much as ten grams of vitamin C daily. This unusually high use of vitamin C caused scientists to conduct studies that have proven its safety to about 5 grams daily. Vitamin C is probably safe even above 5 grams; it's just that there aren't many studies to call on.

I'll cover each issue that concerned people when this use of vitamin C started, just in case you encounter them.

• *Rebound scurvy:* This theory proposed by a physician states that when you stop taking high levels of vitamin C you get scurvy, even though you're still getting the basic level daily, because the body adapts to high levels of vitamin C. This physician presented two cases in which infants got some gum lesions.

Rebound scurvy proved to be a bankrupt notion. Not only could it not be reproduced clinically, but the original cases were shown to have had other causes. In short, our body doesn't adapt to high levels of vitamin C.

• *Kidney stones:* Some kidney stones are crystals of calcium oxalate. Physicians often mistakenly tell their patients who have kidney stones forming to stop taking calcium and extra vitamin C. The reason they implicate vitamin C is because a byproduct of its metabolism is oxalic acid, which with calcium forms calcium oxalate.

Clinicians immediately started giving people who were forming kidney stones large amounts of vitamin C to see if they'd excrete more oxalic acid. Oxalic acid output in these people simply remained the same. Since then, scientists have learned that kidney stone formation isn't related to vitamin C, its metabolism, or even calcium. Consequently, another safety issue about vitamin C went up in smoke. The best thing to do if you're a "stone former" is to drink lots of water.

• *Fetal toxicity:* Some people felt that excess vitamin-C intake by pregnant women could cause either deformities or fetal stress. Both notions were settled by studies showing that there's no correlation. Indeed, pregnant women not getting enough vitamin C put their developing infants at serious risk, as can be seen in the increased incidence of childhood brain tumors in these infants.

• *Gout:* Some research indicates that vitamin C, at about 4 grams daily, increases uric acid levels in the blood. This suggests an upper limit of 4 grams for people whose uric acid is already high or who have gout.

• *Interaction with other nutrients:* Vitamin C can interact with other vitamins and minerals, so it was thought that people who use large amounts of vitamin C could run the risk of other deficiencies. Research soon set this notion aside. The bottom line of all this research is that vitamin C is safe at 5 to 10 grams daily. It's probably even safe above that level. However, such large loads of vitamin C can cause diarrhea. Therefore, go slowly if you decide to use a lot of vitamin C, and don't take it all at once.

BASIC NEEDS DIET

Five servings of fruits and vegetables daily will generally supply 100 milligrams of vitamin C. I get that value by assuming you'll eat three servings of vitamin-C-rich vegetables or fruit, such as broccoli, tomatoes, green or red peppers, an orange, grapefruit, strawberries, or cantaloupe. These fruits and vegetables contain up to 50 milligrams of vitamin C per serving, on average. In addition, other fruits and vegetables, including potatoes and rice, contain from 15 to 50 milligrams per serving, on average. So if you follow the Longevity Diet, you'll meet your 100-milligram need with room to spare. Table 2.3 at the end of this chapter lists the best sources of vitamin C.

BEYOND BASIC NEEDS: SUPPLEMENTS

First I'd like to urge you to reduce the need for additional vitamin C imposed by lifestyle and poor health habits. You should begin by recognizing what causes increased need for vitamin C, so you can meet increased need by taking extra vitamin C or reduce it so you don't need any extra.

- Don't eat processed meats. Read ingredient lists. If you see "nitrate" or "nitrite" on a food product, put it back on the shelf. Have one vitamin-C-rich food or a vitamin C supplement at each meal.

- Know your water supply. Get an analysis. If it contains nitrates, drink bottled water or install a home purifier that removes them.

- Don't smoke. If you work, commute, or live in a city or urban setting, get an extra 250 milligrams of vitamin C daily.

- Avoid physical stress by using common sense. Dress warmly in cold weather. Keep your house warm or wear a sweater. Don't work to exhaustion. When extra-heavy activity is required, take extra vitamin C.

- When emotional stress occurs, strive for 500 milligrams of vitamin C daily.

- If you have a chronic health problem, such as bleeding gums or respiratory problems, if you catch colds easily, become infected easily when scratched or cut, have allergies, or are often tired and fatigued, you may need extra vitamin C. It's safer to take more vitamin C than be sorry you didn't.

SHOULD I TAKE SUPPLEMENTAL VITAMIN C?

I get this question more than any other. I also find more "closet" vitamin-C users than any other "closet" user supplement.

A "closet" user is a nutrition or dietetic educator who teaches people they get all the vitamins they need from a balanced diet, but then supplements his or her own diet with up to 500 milligrams of vitamin C daily. That's far more than you could get from dietary sources unless you made a serious effort every day.

In my opinion, 100 milligrams of vitamin C is a basic amount. I believe most people need about 500 milligrams of vitamin C daily from food and as supplements. Evidence to support your need for extra vitamin C keeps growing, and no evidence accumulates to dispute it.

In view of the historical perspective and the role of bioflavonoids, I believe any vitamin C supplement should contain a liberal amount of bioflavonoids. Too little is known about these materials to offer any quantitative advice but, in my opinion, a 500-milligram vitamin C tablet should include about 100 milligrams of bioflavonoids.

TO GET 100 MILLIGRAMS OF VITAMIN C DAILY

- Eat one serving of 50 milligrams or greater of a vitamin-C-rich fruit, vegetable, or fruit juice daily.

- Have five servings of fruit or vegetables daily.

GETTING MORE THAN 100 MILLIGRAMS OF VITAMIN C DAILY

- Eat or drink fruits or fruit juices extra rich in vitamin C, such as citrus fruits. Count each extra serving as 50 milligrams.

- A 500-milligram vitamin C-supplement should contain bioflavonoids and release the vitamin C slowly. If you're going to supplement with vitamin C, take 500 milligrams daily.

I believe the evidence that vitamin C is an important protector is overwhelming. I also know that the amount we need for this purpose isn't clear, so I take at least 500 milligrams of vitamin C daily as a sustained-release supplement that also contains 120 milligrams of bioflavonoids.

TABLE 2.3

Best Fruit, Vegetable, and Juice Sources of Vitamin C

	Amount of vitamin C, in milligrams
FRUITS	
50 or More Milligrams Vitamin C per Serving*	
Acerola	1,644
Papaya	188
Guava	165
Pomelo	116
Black currants	101
Strawberries	85
Longans	84
Orange, navel	80
Kiwi fruit	75
Lychees	72
Jujube	69
Cantaloupe	68
Orange, valencia	57
Mango	57
Sugar apple	56
Elderberries	52
Mulberries	51
20 to 50 Milligrams Vitamin C per Serving	
Grapefruit	47
Pitanga	46
Sapote	45
Mandarin orange	43
Gooseberries	42
Lemon	31
Breadfruit	28
Carambola	27
Honeydew melon	27
Tangerine	26
Sapodilla	25

Currants (red & white)	23
Soursop	23
Rose apple	22
Casaba melon	21
Lime	20

10 to 20 Milligrams Vitamin C per Serving

Custard apple	19
Persimmon	17
Plantain	17
Blackberries	15
Raspberries	15
Watermelon	15
Quince	14
Cranberries	13
Loganberries	12
Pineapple	12
Apricots (3 medium)	11
Banana (medium)	10
Blueberries	10
Java plum	10

VEGETABLES

Pepper (hot)	109
Pepper, sweet red	95
Broccoflower™	75
Pepper, sweet green	64
Brussels sprouts	48
Cassava	48
Broccoli	41
Seaweed (nori)	39
Cauliflower	36
Lotus root	36
Dock	32
Peas	31
Swamp cabbage	31
Sweet potato	28
Kale	27
Parsley	27
Collards	23

Onions	23
Chickory greens	22
Potato	22
Tomato	22
Red cabbage	20
Rutabaga	19
Asparagus	18
Beet greens	18
Green cabbage	18
Mustard greens	18
Garden cress	17
Turnip greens	17
Chinese cabbage	16
Swiss chard	16
Soybeans	15
Spinach	15
Squash (most)	15
Avocado	14
Okra	13
Lima beans	11
Dandelion greens	10
Radish	10

FRESH OR FROZEN JUICES

Acerola	3,872
Orange	124
Lemon	112
Cranberry	108
Grapefruit	94
Tangerine	77
Passion fruit	74
Lime	72
Grape	60
V-8 juice	52
Tomato	33
Pineapple	30

*All food servings are ½ cup or 1 medium fruit or vegetable.
All juice servings are 1 cup.

3

Vitamin E and Tocopherols

"Fleurs de cimetiere," the French way of saying "age spots," sounds so elegant. As we age, these spots appear on the backs of our hands, on our faces, and on other parts of the body. Though you can't see them, they also appear on the internal organs.

Age spots are locations where pigments involving rancid oils, called lipofuscin, have accumulated. French folk wisdom would have it that wheat germ or wheat germ oil prevents age spots. The only nutritional way to prevent the onset of age spots is with vitamin E, and wheat germ oil happens to be the best natural source of vitamin E. So, once more, folk wisdom rings true.

Though this folk wisdom was mostly oriented toward looks, it goes right to the heart of vitamin E's function: preventing the oxidation of essential oils in the body. In this way, vitamin E actually slows the aging process.

Aging toward our maximum life span is normal. By comparison, aging toward a shorter life expectancy is a disease. Call this disease "accelerated aging." Vitamin E is a protector in our fight against accelerated aging. Though vitamin E can't make us young again, it helps us hold fast to the spirit of youth, mentally and physically.

THE CURE FINDS A DISEASE

Before 1970, vitamin E was a cure in search of a disease. The many human functions it protects can be conveniently grouped into an overused comment: "that's part of aging." This grouping includes emphysema, cataracts, bronchial problems, loss of alertness, loss of vision, sensory perception, and response, decline in walking ability, loss of blue-yellow visual sensitivity, and environmental cancers. They're all difficult, if not impossible, to quantify, so they go unstudied in science and are labeled as the catchall "aging."

A common thread connects these "aging" symptoms: cell breakdown from free radicals and superoxides. Vitamin E is an antioxidant that protects all cells in general and nerve cells specifically. It is similar to beta carotene in its method of protection and simply works better than beta carotene in some tissues and parts of the cell. Vitamin E also works with vitamin C and the mineral selenium to protect the polyunsaturated oils, especially the omega-3 oils, from oxidation. You'll read about these protectors in chapter 8.

***

Vitamin E Quiz

Answer yes or no to these questions:

- Are you athletic or do you engage in high output activities, such as running, cycling, swimming, or cross-country skiing?

- Do you eat high-fat processed foods, such as bologna or frankfurters?

- Do you smoke or work in a smoky or fume-filled environment?

- Do you work in, live in, or commute to a metropolitan area?

- Do you or your parents have age spots?

- Have you or your parents suffered a decline in vision?

- If you're a woman, have you ever had cysts in your breasts or has your doctor said you have fibrocystic breast disease?

A yes to any of these questions means you need to know more about vitamin E. After you learn more about its relevance to your personal life, you can decide how much you need.

HOW THE CURE FOUND THE DISEASE

Vitamin E was discovered at the University of California, Berkeley, in 1922. Scientists developed a diet that prevented female rats from reproducing. When they added green, leafy vegetables, the rats reproduced, so they concluded that a factor in these vegetables was necessary for reproduction.

Four years later, Dr. Karl Mason proved that the same diet caused male rats' testicles to degenerate; they couldn't father offspring. When green, leafy vegetables were added to the rats' diet, their testicles remained normal and the males could sire offspring. So the factor had no sexual bias.

At the time, scientists classified newly discovered vitamins alphabetically, so this new factor was called vitamin E. By 1933, it was identified chemically and named tocopherol from two Greek words, *tokos,* which means offspring, and *pherein,* which means to bear. Therefore, tocopherol, or vitamin E, meant "to bear offspring." People have mistakenly related it to sexual capacity ever since.

In 1931 researchers found that vitamin-E deficiency caused muscular dystrophy in rabbits and hamsters. They discovered in 1939 that vitamin-E deficiency led to blood leakage from capillaries and brain hemorrhage in chickens. Inadequate supplies of vitamin E were found in 1949 to cause fragile red blood cells in all animals, producing anemia. In 1960, researchers reported that vitamin-E deficiency caused muscular dystrophy and anemia in monkeys. So by 1960 there was ample evidence that vitamin E was necessary for general good health in animals. But after three years in a study of a vitamin E-deficient diet in human volunteers, no symptoms were observed. Many scientists concluded there wasn't any human need for vitamin E. But luck favors the mind that's prepared.

In 1966 at Columbia Medical School Hospital in New York City, a group of infants became irritable and developed anemia and fluid retention. It was discovered that all these symptoms occurred because their formulas were vitamin-E deficient. When they were given vitamin E, the symptoms cleared up. At last, a human need for vitamin E was found.

Since 1966, other deficiencies have been identified, such as neuropathies and visual sensitivities, in people who don't absorb vitamin E from food. These findings leave no doubt that vitamin E is a required nutrient for humans.

In 1969, the National Academy of Sciences declared vitamin E to be essential in man and animals. They gave it an RDA in the 1969 edition of *Recommended Dietary Allowances.*

WHAT IS VITAMIN E?

Eight materials provide vitamin E activity: four tocopherols and four close cousins, the tocotrienols, all are chemically classified as fats and therefore sparingly soluble in water. In assessing the ability of these materials to restore rats' sexual viability, alpha tocopherol is rated at 100 percent and the other materials range from about 1 percent to 30 percent. All these materials are seed oils. The best source is wheat oil, but they're also found in such seeds as soy, corn, peanuts, walnuts, and others, as well as most vegetables. Seed oils are also found in the flesh of animals that eat these foods. Food sources of vitamin E are summarized at the end of this chapter.

Vitamin E is expressed in terms of alpha tocopherol. We say you need 10 milligrams of alpha-tocopherol activity if you're an adult, and 12 milligrams if you're an infant. It wasn't always this way. In the past, vitamin E was expressed in international units (I.U.). One milligram of alpha tocopherol is 1.625 I.U. of vitamin E. The government doesn't make things easy. In fact, they're in the process of changing it again.

In 1968, the first RDA for vitamin E was 30 I.U. or 18 milligrams. It was subsequently dropped in the next edition of *Recommended Dietary Allowances* to 15 I.U. or about 10 milligrams. In the 1989 edition of *Recommended Dietary Allowances,* vitamin E need is now expressed only as 10 milligrams. These changes were not based so much on need, as on what practical levels are found in the diet.

AGING: MYTH AND PROMISE

Vitamin E increases the average life span of laboratory animals, but not the maximum life span. This means that if the maximum life span of a mouse is one hundred days, and poor environmental conditions reduce it to an average of fifty days, you can increase its life span, perhaps to seventy-five days, by adding more vitamin E to its diet. However, you can't push life expectancy beyond one hundred days with vitamin E, even under optimal conditions. In animals vitamin E slowed the aging processes brought on by some environmental factors, such as bad air, and helped them reach their maximum life span. If vitamin E does this in animals, it works for humans as well, because environmental factors have been proven to have the same effects on us as they do on rats and other experimental animals.

Another experiment deals with a pigment, lipofuscin, that accumulates in central nerve tissues as we age. Lab animals deficient in vitamin E build more age pigment in their nerve tissue than animals with enough vitamin E. As the pigment builds, the ability of animals to perform tasks, such as running a maze, declines. These tasks require both memory and nerve-muscle coordination. Lipofuscin slows both functions: it increases the loss of memory and coordination. Lipofuscin is the nervous system's equivalent of age spots.

We don't know for sure if there's a cause and effect relationship between age spots and aging. Does the age pigment lipofuscin simply accumulate, or does it have an adverse effect on the body's function? Evidence from animal studies would suggest it causes the decline that comes with aging! Proof is slowly mounting that shows the age pigment does, in fact, slow things down in people. It's a sort of sludge that accumulates more rapidly in the absence of vitamin E.

Researchers tested the maze-running ability by feeding animals a diet rich in polyunsaturated fat like ours, but deficient in vitamin E. Other animals were given the same diet supplemented with vitamin E. Animals with vitamin E maintained a good maze-running ability. Animals without vitamin E lost the ability. You'll see later that this loss results from the polyunsaturated fat in nerve tissue not being protected from free-radical attack. Vitamin E is the major protector of these essential oils.

Tumor development is a normal part of aging. The older you are, the more likely you are to have tumors, both cancerous and benign. So the final test is to compare tumor rates in animals with and without vitamin E. Here's another blockbuster: vitamin E slows tumor development, especially of environmental tumors. Environmental tumors are those that accumulate in the aerodigestive tissues, which include the lips, mouth, throat, nasal passages, and lung tissues.

We can raise animals in an environmentally imperfect environment and monitor three clear aging markers. Vitamin E slows each marker down; aging pigment doesn't build as quickly, mental processes remain viable longer, and tumors accumulate more slowly.

The bottom line: Does this protection apply to humans? The answer is a firm yes! By studying vitamin E at the level of each cell, we can learn how it slows aging in humans.

CELL MEMBRANES

We find vitamin E in all cells of the body. In each of our fifty trillion cells, vitamin E is an integral part of the cell membrane. Cell membranes are the first line of defense against toxic agents. They consist of oils, proteins, carbohydrates, and many other materials in an exceedingly complex chemical structure. When the integrity of the membrane is broken, several disastrous problems can develop for the cell. Cell contents can leak out and, at the extreme, can cause the cell to die. Specific cell functions can be changed by things leaking in and out or getting lost, such as the transmission of signals along a nerve cell. Toxins can get in and attack the genetic material in the nucleus, creating the possibility of a mutation leading to a tumor. Other destructive events are possible, but these three examples are enough to make the point: the cell membrane is the first line of defense.

Vitamin E protects the cell membrane from attack by free radicals and superoxides. It is notably protective of the polyunsaturated oils, major components of all cells, especially the nervous system cells. Polyunsaturated oils (chapter 8) are especially vulnerable to attack by free radicals and superoxides because of their chemical structure. Since they are so critical to the structure of biological membranes, a major role of vitamin E is to protect them from destruction.

Vitamin E is an especially good protector because the materials that form between free radicals or superoxides and vitamin E are not toxic themselves. Therefore, vitamin E is a completely safe protector, even after it has been sacrificed and formed a new ''waste'' material.

From what we know, we'd expect vitamin E to protect cells from attack by free radicals and superoxides. Cells that are particularly vulnerable are those exposed to the environment and cells of the nervous system that are especially rich in the polyunsaturated oils, and specifically, the essential oils, such as the omega-3 and omega-6 oils that we'll discuss in chapter 9.

SYNERGY: NATURE'S DEFENSE STRATEGY

The word *synergy* comes from the Greek word *synergos,* meaning ''working together,'' so each partner enhances the effectiveness of the other. The whole is greater than the sum of its parts. Look at it this way: if each member of a synergistic relationship contributes one unit, and they work together, the sum isn't two; it's three or more. That's how vitamins E and C work together and how vitamin E works with an unusual mineral, selenium. They're all antioxidants.

Antioxidants enhance the effect of each other. Each one has a sphere of influence and is found on the cell at a specific location. And like anything that has a sphere of influence, there's an outer zone where its influence becomes less and tapers to nothing. However, if another antioxidant, such as vitamin C or selenium, is nearby and the weak zones overlap, where the weak zone of vitamin E overlaps with either the weak zone of vitamin C or selenium, the overlapping zone becomes a well-protected area; hence, synergism between two nutrients. We're the beneficiary.

The cell membrane and other systems are protected from free radicals and superoxides by these antioxidants. In some cells, such as red blood cells, vitamin E is the only protector. In other cells it's vitamin E and selenium. And in still other cells, the eye lens, for example, vitamins E and C make up the defense force. The more protectors there, the better the defense.

ATHLETES: CELL MEMBRANES

When scientists realized that free radicals and superoxides were blocked by vitamin E, Dr. Al Tappel at the University of California, Davis, conducted a very revealing experiment with athletes.

Tappel knew that when the polyunsaturated fats in cell membranes of the lungs are oxidized, the byproducts of those oxidation reactions can be measured in the exhaled air. So why not have some athletes exercise vigorously near maximum capacity and measure the byproducts before and after giving the athletes extra vitamin E?

The athletes established the level of oxidation byproducts by running at maximum capacity on a treadmill with a breathing device attached to their mouth that recovered the gases they exhaled. Then they were divided into two groups; one group took 1,200 I.U., that's 750 milligrams, of vitamin E, and the other a placebo daily and repeated the treadmill test every day for two weeks. Oxidative byproducts dropped by more than 50 percent in the E-enriched group, depending on what level of maximum capacity they ran. This experiment simply proved that vitamin E protects cell membranes from oxidation. This single experiment did more; it suggested that all the animal studies with vitamin E apply to humans.

This study proves two points: vitamin E prevents oxidative destruction of cell membranes, and people who exercise vigorously should probably strive for higher-than-average levels of vitamin E.

I should point out that there's nothing magical about 1,200 I.U. of vitamin E. It was chosen as a significant but safe excessive amount to establish an effect. I doubt that less than 600 I.U. would have been effective, since the athletes were at maximum activity.

NEUROLOGICAL PROTECTION

Of all tissues, the nervous system is particularly vulnerable to free-radical attack because nerve cells characteristically have a larger amount of polyunsaturated fats than other tissues. In addition, the polyunsaturated fats are critical to the function of the entire tissue and not simply the membrane of each cell. Neuropathies, such as tingling or numbness in fingers and toes, are seen in vitamin-E-deficient adults. These neuropathies are usually accompanied by a loss of coordination, a combination of factors that implicate complete nervous system involvement.

Alcoholics are particularly vulnerable to developing neuropathies. Excessive alcohol consumption causes an increase in the free-radical destruction of vitamin E. Thus, chronic alcoholics usually show a relationship between low vitamin-E levels and nerve damage, even atrophy of the brain. It's a tragic way to prove that the antioxidant effects of vitamin E protect humans much as they do rats.

EYE DEVELOPMENT

The retina of the eye is the most sensitive nerve tissue. Its functions can easily be measured by flashing a light and measuring the impulse generated in the eye. Then, by changing the location of the flash, but not of the eye, you can map the sensitivity of the eye.

In vitamin-E deficiency, the retina loses its visual sensitivity from the center outward. When adequate levels of vitamin E are restored, vision returns slowly but completely in about two years. This slow motion restoration is typical of the slow regeneration of nerve tissue, and the slow movement of vitamin E, which moves with fat in the body because it's an oil and cannot dissolve in water. In contrast, water-soluble vitamin C literally flows with the water, so when it's deficient, restoration comes fast. Recall that the symptoms of scurvy cleared up in a couple of weeks.

CATARACTS

Once scientists recognized that free radicals and superoxides damage tissues, it was a small step to look at cataracts. Cataract formation increases with any effect that produces free radicals; these include smoking, air pollution, and excessive sunlight, which are the big three. It would be logical to expect vitamins E and C and beta carotene to protect against cataracts, because they block free radicals and superoxides.

Most studies show cataract reduction of up to 80 percent when vitamin C and vitamin E are taken together. Vitamin C alone, at about 500 milligrams daily, gains a 50-percent reduction, but adding a little more vitamin E at the same time pushes this rate over 70 percent.

The anatomy of the eye lens probably accounts for this effect. The lens consists of three distinct regions, one of which is especially rich in vitamin C. All cells of the lens have membranes that are rich in vitamin E. Consequently, you'd expect a synergistic effect in the eye between vitamins E and C. Beta carotene is also important in eye protection but doesn't have the same power as vitamins E and C.

EMPHYSEMA

Emphysema is a disease of the air sacs in the lungs. Lung tissues consist of a countless number of microscopic balloons called air sacs. Blood capillaries line each air sac. When we breathe in, an exchange of gases takes place during the instant that the air is in our lungs: the blood in the capillaries takes oxygen from the air and releases the carbon dioxide and other gases it contains. Then when you exhale, the waste gases are released.

Many gases are exchanged in both directions in the process. We know this from the experience of being caught in smoke, from being anesthetized for general surgery, and from the highs experienced by smokers and drug users. We know other gases are released from the lungs by smelling the breath of someone who's been drinking or has recently eaten garlic. From this experience, you know these air sacs are exposed to whatever you breathe and they release the volatile things from the food you eat.

Air sacs are irritated and damaged by some irritating or oxidizing gases in the air. These include ozone, an especially active and corrosive form of oxygen, nitrogen oxides from exhaust fumes, and many other materials ranging from household solvents to toxic gas. If we expose laboratory rats to these fumes, they develop emphysema.

Emphysema is a disease in which the air sacs become enlarged, more specifically inflamed, and lose their ability to stretch when we breathe in and snap back when we breathe out. In short, the enlarged sacs are like a balloon that has lost its elasticity.

Emphysema isn't given much press. At times it has been called a disease of aging. Smokers are especially likely to get emphysema if they don't get cancer first. People who work in smoke or fumes are more likely to get this disease as they age. In fact, about 390,000 people die annually from emphysema or related bronchial tube degeneration. That's more than American battle deaths in World War II.

We all get emphysema to some extent, but not badly enough so it's noticeable. You could probably say we'd all get it if we lived long enough. When emphysema is advanced, it's as serious as losing your legs.

Life with emphysema is a nightmare. You're always out of breath and must always have an oxygen tank nearby in case you get tired out. Many times you can't get enough oxygen to stand up, so people with emphysema often live in a wheelchair.

A fluid called aveolar fluid bathes the air sacs of the lung, the aveoli. Lung tissue contains more vitamin E than most tissues, and the aveolar fluid also contains vitamin E. Some people don't have as much of this protective fluid as they should, and others don't have as much vitamin E in their lung tissues or fluid as normal. For example, smokers have less of both. Either situation makes them more susceptible to emphysema.

Vitamin E helps protect us from emphysema in the aveolar fluid and the cells of the air sacs. People who get respiratory illnesses easily, smoke, or work in fumes or polluted air can insure their health by making sure they get optimum amounts of vitamin E. We'll all get emphysema as we grow older, but vitamin E slows down the rate of development.

CANCER PROTECTION: WHY?

Animal studies prove vitamin E protects against cancer in most tissues. Researchers simply feed animals differing levels of vitamin E and apply known cancer-causing materials to various parts of their bodies. When they do this, vitamin E protects against most cancer-causing chemicals, especially those that involve free radicals or superoxides, and protects membranes, such as lungs and aerodigestive tissues.

Indeed, scientists have placed animals in noxious environments of chemicals found in auto exhaust and other toxic pollutants. Not only do these poor animals live longer when given more vitamin E, but cancer is reduced in proportion. In fact, the incidence of all types of tumors declines.

We would also expect there to be less cancer because of vitamin E's ability to block nitrosamine formation. Nitrosamines are the same cancer-causing agents you learned about in chapter 2, on vitamin C. They're produced in our body from nitrates and nitrites in the diet. Vitamin E blocks nitrosamine development in a manner similar to the way in which vitamin C blocks it, except vitamin E works in fatty systems and tissues because it's a fat. Vitamin C, being a carbohydrate and water soluble, works in watery systems. Vitamin E should reduce cancer formation, especially in parts of the digestive system where there is a lot of fatty tissue and nitrates are converted to nitrosamines (the stomach is the prime candidate).

Vitamin E also contributes to cancer prevention indirectly because it's necessary for a strong immune system. As a component of healthy cell membranes, vitamin E is essential to all cells, including those that attack cancer cells, so we'd expect vitamin E to contribute to a reduction of all cancers.

HOW TO PROVE A VITAMIN E CONNECTION

Unlike the case of beta carotene, it's difficult to measure the amount of vitamin E in an individual's diet, but it's related to the fats and oils in our diet. Since 1850, the percentage of calories we get from fat has increased from 13 percent to over 40 percent at present. Most of this fat is from animals as meat and from dairy products. Since vitamin E comes from diverse vegetable foods, we can't conclude that more fat means more vitamin E. In fact, it's quite likely to be the opposite. Scientists overcome relating the abundance of fat to vitamin E by going directly to blood samples. Blood levels of vitamin E are the best measure because they cut through all the pitfalls of dietary analysis. So most of us are getting vitamin E from diverse sources. This forces scientists to search for the cancer connection using blood analyses.

In one technique, called "prospective," blood is repeatedly taken from a group of people over time and frozen for later analysis. As the group ages and dies, various aspects of the members' blood chemistry can be evaluated. This technique is also useful in the light of new discoveries. For example, suppose we find that some compound, call it X, in the blood prevents a rare disease. We can return to the frozen samples and see if it existed in them, whether its presence or absence was affected by aging or other factors noted when the blood samples were taken.

A second technique, known as "retrospective," is to simply freeze blood from people when they are diagnosed with cancer and make the samples available to epidemiologists who later think they can find a relationship to some blood component. This also provides a good way of comparing new findings to cases from the past. If the findings are solid, they should stand up to various tests. Scientists have done both techniques with vitamin E, and theory stands up to their expectations.

CANCER PROTECTION: VITAMIN E PASSES

Scientists in Finland followed a group of people for ten years and are still following them. In this Finnish prospective study, frozen blood samples can be compared and reexamined in the light of other scientific discoveries.

In the United States and other countries, the National Institutes of Health keep frozen blood samples. These samples can be used retrospectively to compare vitamin-E levels to various types of cancer. The results of several studies in the United States, Finland, and England produced several findings:

- Prospective studies have shown a general reduction of all cancers, specifically breast, stomach, and intestinal cancer, and a clear trend in reducing lung cancer related to high vitamin-E levels in the blood.
- Retrospective studies show a clear reduction of lung and breast cancer, and general reduction trends in other cancers tied to higher vitamin-E blood levels.
- Combination studies in which both prospective and retrospective techniques were used confirmed the findings of fewer cases of aerodigestive cancer (lips, mouth, nose, esophagus, etc.) with increased blood levels of vitamin E. They also confirmed reduced rates of lung and stomach cancer if vitamin E was present in the blood at higher levels.
- A prospective study of the rate of breast cancer in women showed that low blood levels of vitamin E and selenium increase the risk of breast cancer ten times over normal. This

is an outstanding conclusion, since it suggests that vitamins C and E work together in breast cancer prevention.

From these studies the relationship is very clear: low blood levels of vitamin E increase the risk of cancer. Your risk of cancer is about twice as great if you have low vitamin-E levels in your blood and about ten times as great if both vitamin-E and selenium levels in the blood are low.

There can no longer be any doubt that dietary vitamin E reduces the risk of cancer. Since vitamin E prevents cancer in general, and since the appearance of tumors is a sign of aging, it would follow that vitamin E reduces the rate of aging. So it appears that French folk wisdom is correct: slow cemetery flowers and you live longer.

FIBROCYSTIC BREAST DISEASE

Fibrous cysts form in the breasts of many women. A cystic breast feels as if it contains a few grains of sand and sometimes as if it's loaded with sand. The breast is sensitive and usually hurts in proportion to the number of cysts. These granules or fibrous cysts, as they are more correctly called, often, but not always, wax and wane with the menstrual cycles. About 10 percent of women start with fibrocystic disease before age twenty-one, and some scientists estimate that by age seventy, 90 percent of women will have had breast cysts sometime during their lives. Should we say, "It's part of aging"?

Experts don't seem to agree that women who get these cysts are more likely to get breast cancer. The same experts point out that women who have fibrocystic breast disease are more likely to survive cancer; probably because they watch themselves more closely and catch the cancer early.

Though not an expert, I conclude from the scientific literature that fibrocystic breast disease is not a clearly understood disease. In general, the experts agree that the cysts are "dysplased cells" and subject to hormonal influence. However, there isn't much agreement on details. The disease first appeared in 1828 as Cooper's Disease and has been described in various ways ever since.

In 1972, scientists from Mt. Sinai Hospital in New York reported positive results on a few women who took vitamin E for fibrocystic breast disease. This report was quickly followed by a larger double-blind study in which about 70 percent of the women improved noticeably. Response varied from a reduction in tenderness in all of them, to complete disappearance of cysts in about 16 percent. (In a double-blind study, neither those giving nor those receiving the medication know if it's medication or a placebo.)

These studies have been followed by others with similarly mixed results. There always seems to be a reduction in discomfort, and some cysts disappear in some women. These results verify that fibrocystic breast disease is not a single or a simple disease.

One certainty emerged from these studies. Women who took the high levels of vitamin E had changes in the byproducts of hormone metabolism in their urine. This is important because of two relationships. Vitamin E has a good correlation with the prevention of breast cancer. A number of studies show that women with low blood levels of vitamin E are more prone to get breast cancer. Breast cancer risk increases with dietary and body fat, but it is also related to the metabolites of hormones. Albeit tenuous, the vitamin E to female hormone relationship is the subject of active research.

A second relationship was observed anecdotally in PMS (premenstrual syndrome). PMS is at various times described as a disease and at other times as a variation of normal for some women. At one meeting of the American College of Nutrition, an organization of physicians and other health professionals who practice and conduct research in nutrition, a paper was presented on PMS showing how confusing the results of nutritional studies on it always turned out. So I asked the presentor the most naive question of all: "Well, doctor, have you ever found anything in nutrition that works consistently in a double-blind study?"

"Vitamin E" was her unabashed reply. These results have never been published! I think the investigator wants to do more studies so the results leave no room for doubt.

NUTRIENT VERSUS DRUG

Results on PMS and fibrocystic breast disease require 600 I.U. or 400 milligrams of vitamin E daily all the time. You don't get 400 milligrams of vitamin E from your diet unless it includes a dose of wheat germ oil. The RDA for vitamin E is 10 milligrams, so 400 milligrams is forty times the RDA. You've got to seek out a vitamin-E supplement to get that much and take it daily. Is it a drug when used under those conditions even though it's sold as a vitamin? I can say without hesitation that vitamin E is safe at levels over 1,000 milligrams daily, so 400 milligrams is surely safe. I don't believe it should be treated as a drug.

VITAMIN E AND HEART DISEASE

In the 1950s and 1960s, two physicians from Canada, Dr. Wilfred E. Shute and his brother, treated heart disease patients with massive amounts of vitamin E. The outstanding results they obtained could never be either achieved again or repeated in clinical trials. But, like many well-intentioned zealots, they created a debate about the effect of vitamin E on arterial plaque—a mound of lipid material, smooth muscle cells, and calcium that accumulates in the inner artery wall—that still persists over thirty years later.

As often happens in science, debate starts research and research leads to new findings. From the Shute brothers' debate, scientists learned that vitamin E increases high-density lipoprotein (HDL) cholesterol. Higher HDL amounts in the blood reduce the risk of heart disease in everyone. So even if the Shutes were wrong, they acted as catalysts for some important research.

Blood cholesterol is divided into several fractions, but for assessing risk, only two numbers are necessary: total cholesterol and HDL cholesterol.

HDL cholesterol is ''good'' cholesterol because it represents the fraction of cholesterol being swept up from the arterial sludge for elimination. Consequently, scientists assess risk by taking the ratio of total cholesterol to HDL cholesterol.

Average risk is a total cholesterol to HDL ratio of about five, and three or less is considered excellent. In this case, the lower your grade is, the better you are; the higher grade, above five, means you should do something right away to get it down. See a cardiologist!

In settling the Shute debate, some researchers found that about 30 milligrams of vitamin E daily helps to boost HDL cholesterol. It may even elevate total cholesterol slightly, because the HDL fraction is increasing. But a slight elevation doesn't matter, because it's in the HDL fraction.

Reducing risk of heart disease involves more than taking extra vitamin E. It starts with a low-fat, high-fiber diet, good lifestyle, and correct exercise. So while I encourage everyone to get vitamin E, I also counsel that it should be one small part of a total program.

SAFETY OF VITAMIN E

Dr. Lawrence Machlin and his colleagues at the Cornell Medical School summarized the vitamin-E safety issue clearly. In studies where people took from 600 I.U. up to 3,200 I.U. of vitamin E daily—that's 400 to 2,000 milligrams—they had no negative side effects at all. There's one minor caution, however. Vitamin E interacts with vitamin K, which is necessary for healthy blood clotting. People who are deficient in vitamin K or are on medication to prevent blood clotting should only take these very high levels of vitamin E *under medical guidance*. However, for normal folks, Dr. Machlin's research proved that levels of vitamin E up to 3,200 I.U.s a day are safe.

This segues nicely into how much we need, how much we get, and where we get it from.

HOW MUCH VITAMIN E?

In 1968, the RDA was set at 30 I.U. or 18 milligrams; five years later it was dropped to 15 I.U. or 9 milligrams. In 1989, it was set at 16 I.U. or 10 milligrams for adults. Did people change? No, they didn't! These changes are an example of what happens when things are done by committees that must deal with symptoms of deficiency and whose objectives aren't always explained to the public. Since the 1989 edition of *Recommended Dietary Allowances* went to press, some controversy led to a lawsuit, so the confusion will continue for the foreseeable future.

When the first RDA for vitamin E was published, in 1968, there were no known symptoms of deficiency, except in some rare cases of premature infants. Symptoms of vitamin-E deficiency are almost impossible to develop. They only occur in people who don't absorb fat because of serious intestinal disorders. Even then, they only occur rarely. Dieticians quickly pointed out to the RDA committee that most people only get about 15 I.U. or 9 milligrams in their diet. Well, the committee reasoned, if there are "no symptoms," then why not reduce the RDA to 15 I.U.; so in 1973 they did.

However, vitamin E protects average people against cataracts, cancer, and neurological symptoms and slows aging. So, in my opinion, that protective level is what we need for optimum health. We can identify how much the average person needs for this level of protection.

Blood levels that seem to reduce the risk of cancer or cataracts to zero require 60 to 100 I.U. of vitamin E daily; that's about 40 to 60 milligrams daily. So we can strike an average at 50 milligrams. If you accept the HDL cholesterol level as more appropriate, you'll settle for 30 to 50 I.U., say 40 I.U., or about 25 milligrams of vitamin E daily.

Now we're left with a dilemma: do we follow the RDA of 10 milligrams of vitamin E for average adults established by a U.S. government committee to prevent overt symptoms, or do we take 50 milligrams of vitamin E, which experts say we need for optimum health to prevent diseases of aging?

Both groups are correct, and you've got to make your own decision; all I can do is help you see the difference.

• RDA committees must be concerned with symptoms of overt disease and body pools. Body pools are like the vitamin-C reservoir for any nutrient. There are no overt symptoms of vitamin-E deficiency at 5 to 10 milligrams (15 I.U.) daily and the body pool is satisfactory. That's the government's responsibility, and they've done a good job! So they're correct in setting the RDAs.

• Optimum health deals with protection from cancer, emphysema, and cataracts. These are not subject to quantitative evaluation and they probably won't be until we approach the year 2050. So, at this time, we can say a certain blood level seems to be protective against these diseases, and to maintain that blood level an adult needs about 50 milligrams of vitamin E daily. Children probably need a proportionate amount of vitamin E.

• PMS and fibrocystic breast disease are unclear conditions at best. Four hundred milligrams of vitamin E daily helps alleviate the symptoms of these problems. You can't get 400 milligrams of vitamin E daily from a practical diet and must rely on the use of food supplements. Though some people would claim that 400 milligrams of vitamin E is a drug, I disagree. Vitamin E is different from other nutrients, and though 400 milligrams is forty times the

RDA, it's still not a drug. However, that's not correct for all nutrients, so don't apply this vitamin-E thinking to other nutrients.

I strive for 50 milligrams daily through diet and sensible supplementation! I've never accepted ''satisfactory'' as the standard for my health or in other aspects of my life. Nutrition is one of the few aspects we can control; I don't leave it to chance.

Inspect the amounts of vitamin E in foods on table 3.1, and you will realize that there are a few good sources of vitamin E.

TABLE 3.1

Vitamin E Content of Foods

Foods	Vitamin E, in Milligrams

Fats and Oils
(Serving size is one tablespoon)

Foods	Vitamin E, in Milligrams
Wheat germ oil	20
Sunflower oil	6
Safflower oil	5
Cottonseed oil	5
Almond oil	5
Corn oil	3
Olive oil	2
Peanut oil	2
Canola oil	3

Other oils provide about 0.5 milligrams per serving.

Nuts and Seeds
(Serving size is one ounce)

Foods	Vitamin E, in Milligrams
Almonds, dried	7
Almonds, oil-roasted	2
Brazil nuts, dried	2
Hazelnuts, dried	7
Peanuts, dried	3
Peanut butter	6
Pistachios	2

Other nuts provide about 0.5 milligrams per ounce.

Cereals
(Serving size is one ounce)

Oatmeal	1
Cornmeal	1
Wheat cereal (whole wheat)	1

Unprocessed cereals provide about 0.5 milligrams per serving. Highly processed cereals provide considerably less.

Baked Goods and Confections

Apple pie, 1/8 pie	7
Blueberry pie, 1/8 pie	7
Pound cake, 3 1/2 ounce	3
Chocolate bar	2
Chocolate cookie, 1	2

Spreads
(All servings are 1 tablespoon)

Margarine	
Mazola, regular or unsalted	8
Mazola, diet	3
Mustard	1
Mayonnaise	
Hellmann's	11
Soybean	3
Peanut butter, Skippy	2

Other spreads provide about 0.5 milligrams per tablespoon.

Grain Products
(Serving size is 1 cup)

Whole-wheat bread (2 slices)	1
Macaroni	1
Spaghetti	1
Wheat germ	1

Other grain products provide about 0.5 milligrams per serving.

Fruits

Mango, 1 medium	2
Apple, medium with skin	1

Other fruits provide less than 0.5 milligrams per serving.

Vegetables
(All servings ½ cup unless specified)

Asparagus, 4 spears	1
Avocado, 1 medium	2
Sweet potato, 1 medium	6

No other vegetables provide one gram of vitamin E.

Fish, Meat, Poultry
(All servings are 3½ ounces)

Chicken, turkey, most fowl	1
Salmon and oily fish	2
Shrimp, scallops, shellfish	3
Beef liver	1

Other meats and nonoily fish provide about 0.5 milligrams per serving.

If you want to get 50 milligrams of vitamin E daily, you will need to take a supplement that contains at least 30 milligrams, and you'd be better off taking one that provides 40 milligrams. One advantage of taking extra vitamin E is that it is retained by your body. Therefore, if you took a 400-I.U. supplement or 240 milligrams once weekly, that would maintain a running average of about 50 milligrams daily if you follow the Longevity Diet. The Longevity Diet will keep you within the RDA but cannot provide 50 milligrams daily. You must use a vitamin-E supplement to get 50 milligrams of vitamin E daily. And since almost all of the most concentrated sources of vitamin E are very high in calories, a vitamin-E supplement will more easily fit into your calorie limits.

Selenium

By A.D. 100, people in parts of China, Siberia, and Russia had learned to brew and drink a therapeutic tea from the leaves of a plant found in all these areas to cure a debilitating form of arthritis in children, which would otherwise have left them crippled for life.

I was present when a friend, who had recently returned from China, discussed the disease. My friend, Dr. Julian Spallholz, flashed a slide of an X ray on the screen. A visiting pediatrician exclaimed, "It's a perfect example of rheumatoid arthritis in a child." The next slide was the X ray of a normal hand, the pediatrician noted. Imagine his surprise when Dr. Spallholz said, "No, they're the same hand before and after the treatment with the tea."

Marco Polo's journal of 1298 refers to a plant in Sinkiang, China, as a poisonous plant, which if eaten [by horses] has the effect of causing the hooves of the animals to drop off. Marco Polo's journal was really the recollections of his journey through China some twenty years previously. This effect of a plant on horses was so remarkable that Polo remembered it twenty years later. The plant has a similar effect on people, except their nails fall off, their hair falls out, and their teeth rot.

These two vignettes illustrate the two faces of the trace element selenium. Selenium is required for our health, but too much of it can be deadly.

WHAT IS SELENIUM?

Selenium is a mineral element whose RDA is set at 70 micrograms. A microgram is a millionth of a gram; 70 micrograms can fit on the period at the end of this sentence, with about 90 percent of the period left open. So, to say selenium is an essential trace mineral seems to define the word *trace*.

Selenium, discovered in 1817, was named after the moon (*selene* in Greek). It is found in many forms, only one of which is important in nutrition. Selenium isn't very abundant. Some soils have very low selenium levels, and food grown in that soil has none. Selenium-deficiency diseases, such as Kaschin-Beck disease, occur in the Shanxi province of China, where the soil is deficient in selenium. Plants called "indicator plants" grow only where selenium is found in the soil and accumulate selenium in their leaves. People from areas with selenium-deficient soil used leaves from the indicator plants to therapeutically correct selenium-deficiency diseases. That's how people cured Kaschin-Beck disease long ago.

In the Dakotas, where the soil contains sufficient selenium, the same indicator plant is called "locoweed." Locoweed brings death to any animal that eats just one, because with the abundant selenium in the soil, the plant becomes toxic with excess selenium. Before the hapless animal dies, it acts crazy with the "blind staggers"; hence the name "locoweed."

During the 1980s in California, the Kesterton Wildlife Refuge was poisoned by selenium that drained into its marshes. Selenium leached from the soil into irrigation water that flowed into the refuge. Clearly, selenium is a mineral that has two faces.

> ### Selenium Quiz

Answer yes or no to these questions:

- Have you or any blood relative had juvenile rheumatoid arthritis?

- Is there a history of cancer in your family?

- Have you or any blood relative ever suffered from muscular weakness or been diagnosed with cardiomyopathy?

- Do you live in, work in, or commute to a city environment?

A yes answer to any of these questions says you should invest a little time in learning about selenium. Though it's not likely you would ever be seriously deficient in selenium, you should know your options.

SELENIUM: THE NUTRIENT

Selenium is unique among the nutrients. The symptom of selenium deficiency in very young children, Kaschin-Beck disease, which appears as a form of rheumatoid arthritis, results from a selenium deficiency in the mother before conception and during pregnancy. Though the mother had no symptoms when pregnant, the newborn child has the disease, which can be eliminated with selenium supplements.

Selenium deficiency after early childhood is characterized by severe pain and weakness of the muscles. In areas where the soil is selenium deficient, as in parts of China, and people eat only locally grown food, serious heart muscle weakness, called cardiomyopathy, develops in adults from longstanding selenium deficiency. Untreated cardiomyopathy is fatal. When it's caused by selenium deficiency, it can be cured with supplements. But if it progresses too long, it can't be reversed.

In North America, the food system is sufficiently varied so that everyone gets a basic level of selenium. Selenium deficiency in the United States and Canada has only appeared in people being fed artificially for a long time with a solution that contained no selenium. In these special cases, the muscular weakness and pain are cleared by adding selenium to the feeding solution. Nowadays, these total parenteral nutrition solutions contain selenium and the problem has been eliminated.

When a person is deficient in both selenium and vitamin E, liver degeneration develops. Although liver failure isn't a deficiency symptom of either nutrient alone, it illustrates how these two nutrients work together. This selenium-vitamin E cooperative protection, called a synergistic effect, will surface again when we explore the protective role of selenium.

By using knowledge gained from artificial feeding, animal studies, and the unique biochemistry of an enzyme that uses selenium, scientists developed a selenium RDA. The biochemistry of selenium has allowed scientists to identify an upper limit at which it becomes unsafe, so we can avoid the dangers of selenium's toxic dark side.

Unlike many other nutrients, selenium is a protector at or slightly above its RDA level. To get a feeling for its protector role, we need to understand its biochemical function.

Most of our fifty trillion cells and our blood have an enzyme called glutathione peroxidase that breaks down natural toxins called peroxides. These peroxides work like those used to bleach hair or remove stains from clothing. Peroxides produce free radicals that are destructive, and the peroxides themselves can destroy body cells and cell components. Glutathione peroxidase, like all enzymes, is a protein and uses a helper called glutathione in its peroxide-destroying task, hence the name, glutathione peroxidase. The glutathione helper requires selenium.

Glutathione peroxidase is essential in many body processes and is found in the blood. For example, it is required in prostaglandin production—prostaglandins are minute amounts of hormonelike chemicals involved in practically every bodily function—so it can indirectly influence inflammation, high blood pressure, the immune system, and other body systems.

Since selenium is required by an enzyme that helps produce the prostaglandins, it's possible that selenium deficiency allows inflammation to run amok. Kaschin-Beck disease appears in children because they're selenium deficient at birth and particularly sensitive to inflammation. In chapter 8 you'll learn about the prostaglandins and how they control inflammation.

The amount of glutathione peroxidase in blood is easily measured by its ability to destroy the kind of peroxide you buy in the store. This method along with feeding studies is used to find the dietary level of selenium the body needs to build a maximum level of the enzyme. Also, this method along with feeding studies is how scientists established the RDA for selenium.

However, destruction of peroxides suggested more than muscle weakness to many scientists. Peroxides are superoxides; that is, they produce and form free radicals easily. Free radicals and superoxides destroy delicate cell membranes, and other cell components, and the byproducts of destructive oxidation can be toxic.

A breached cell membrane opens a cell to attack by cancer-causing agents. Worse yet, a free radical could change a cell's genetic material and convert it to a precancerous cell. So it makes sense that if selenium prevents this conversion to a cancer cell, it's a protector as well as a nutrient.

Since the antioxidant function of selenium was so well established, Clement Ip of the Rosewell Park Memorial Institute in Buffalo, New York, an institute devoted to cancer research, wanted to see if there was a cancer connection. He collected and interpreted worldwide statistics on breast and colon cancer. He compared mortality rates from breast and colon cancer worldwide and compared the rate with the level of selenium in the diet. He reached a startling conclusion: High levels of dietary fat and low levels of dietary selenium are associated with high rates of breast and colon cancer. We've known about the fat association for a long time, but the selenium connection was new. So he sought to study the connection between fat and selenium in breast cancer in rats.

He fed a high-fat diet consisting mostly of polyunsaturated fats (like our diet) to rats; then he gave them an agent that causes breast cancer. If he then supplemented the rats' diet with selenium, only half as many tumors developed. He realized that he was clearly dealing with a protective effect. The next step was to find out what else was involved. He knew that a diet high in polyunsaturated fat requires extra vitamin E to protect the fat.

Ip's next experiment included adding supplemental vitamin E. He added it with and without selenium. Adding vitamin E until it reaches adequate blood levels reduces tumors by about 15 percent. Add selenium to vitamin E, and tumors drop below 50 percent. If you give the animals only excess vitamin E, the rate of tumor development drops by 30 percent. Include adequate selenium with excess vitamin E, and incidence of tumors drops by 60 percent! Clearly, vitamin E and selenium work together as protectors! The greatest effect requires higher than RDA, but not excessive dietary levels of vitamin E and selenium.

In a further experiment, Ip showed that selenium and vitamin E work together as protectors. He started the animals on a diet supplemented with selenium and added vitamin E two days before he introduced the cancer-causing chemical. He then continued the protectors in one group for two days after and in another group for twenty-four days after the cancer-causing agent was added. He gave another group the cancer-causing agent two days before he supplemented their diet with selenium and vitamin E. To summarize Ip's study: The control group that received no vitamin E or selenium had 100 percent of the expected tumors. The group that had only selenium had 64 percent of the tumors anticipated. The group receiving the protectors for two extra days had a 58-percent tumor rate, while the group that had the protectors for twenty-four days had 32 percent of the expected tumors. When the cancer-causing agent was added two days before the protectors, the tumor rate was 35 percent of normal. Clement Ip brought theory and practice to the same focus. Selenium is a protector mineral that works with vitamin E. He confirmed what epidemiology has proven time and again, that high-fat diets promote cancer. Therefore, they require more vitamin E and selenium.

HUMAN PROTECTION FROM CANCER

Epidemiologists started their search for the human protective effect in Finland. Finland is a country where most of the soil is selenium deficient, so you'd expect to find more people with low body levels of selenium than in areas of sufficient soil selenium. Finland also keeps excellent health records.

Finnish results agreed with Ip's. Low blood levels of selenium carried a higher risk of cancer. Similar findings have since been made in the United States, Sweden, and China. Theory, animal studies, and human epidemiology all agree: selenium is a cancer protector, and it works best with vitamin E.

Selenium protects against breast cancer, colon cancer, epithelial cancer—membranes of the mouth, lungs, stomach, and so on— esophageal cancer, and skin cancer. Protection by selenium also involves vitamin E, and recent findings have shown that it works with carotenoids, specifically beta carotene. These findings prove a point: ''In nutrition, teamwork is essential.''

Selenium's function as an antioxidant is not the complete story. Its part with vitamin E in the antioxidant story probably accounts for much of its protection. However, there are nagging bits and pieces of research data that suggest several other functions for selenium.

The fact that selenium protects better if it is added before exposure to cancer-causing agents suggests that it boosts other systems. Some scientists suggest selenium is essential for the immune system. Indeed, glutathione peroxidase is involved in prostaglandin synthesis, and when prostaglandins go awry, the immune system runs amok.

A prostaglandin connection implicates another nutrient, vitamin C. Vitamin C regenerates glutathione peroxidase after it has been deactivated by acting on the prostaglandins. Therefore, a connection between selenium and vitamin C probably exists that has fallen through the "research cracks." It's another example of teamwork that needs to be understood.

Japanese researchers found different selenium tissue levels among different families. This is surprising since the Japanese are a homogeneous people, and within any region their diets are very similar. It brings us full circle to Kaschin-Beck disease in which selenium deficiency shows up in offspring. It all suggests that some people handle dietary selenium better than others.

Look at it this way. There's a given level of selenium in the soil that dictates the level of selenium in food grown in that soil. Because most plants are passive to selenium, they don't accumulate selenium over what's delivered in the soil, so everyone who eats those plants should have the same blood level of selenium. But some people's bodies extract more selenium from food and use it more efficiently than others, so their selenium blood levels are higher. There are a lot of loose ends we need to tighten up by more research.

TOXICITY: ANOTHER FACE OF SELENIUM

Human selenium toxicity is not well understood. Humans consuming just 5 milligrams of selenium daily from food have garlic breath, are very listless and nervous, and lose their fingernails and hair. One milligram daily produces deformed nails and the distinctive garliclike odor that accompanies selenium toxicity. The garlic odor is the byproduct of selenium metabolism in our body. It's a sure sign you're getting too much selenium. Hair and nail loss are minor symptoms; others include nerve disorders, vomiting, and total fatigue.

Obviously selenium toxicity is something to avoid. Not surprisingly, the symptoms suggest that an excess of selenium attacks many systems, including the central nervous system. Scientists have many years of research ahead to work out how and why selenium is toxic at high levels. But at this point, we're able to set some limits to how much is safe.

A safe upper limit of selenium from food is about 300 micrograms per day. There's no need for an average adult to get more than that. That's 0.3 milligrams. Three hundred micrograms still doesn't cover the period at the end of this sentence. We're still in the trace range.

HOW MUCH SELENIUM?

Selenium has an RDA for adults of 50 to 70 micrograms and 75 micrograms for pregnant and nursing women. At that daily level, the enzyme systems that depend on selenium will be fully functioning. Adding more selenium won't make the enzymes any more effective; however, selenium's protector role requires more than the RDA.

Evidence suggests that 90 to 100 micrograms of selenium daily meet its protector need when there are adequate amounts of vitamin E, but it's just as important to get sufficient vitamin E at the same time. Indeed, the protector requirement for selenium is co-dependent on vitamin E. Since vitamin E is safe at even forty times the RDA, it's best to get lots of vitamin E and settle on about 100 to 150 micrograms of selenium. Unlike most antioxidants, more selenium is not necessarily better. After a careful review of toxicity information, it's been determined that 1 milligram daily for six or more months is definitely toxic, even if the symptoms seem mild. Therefore, let 300 micrograms be the upper limit of your daily intake.

DIETARY SELENIUM

Table 4.1 summarizes the most readily available food sources of selenium. The Longevity Diet in chapter 15 provides more than enough selenium.

TABLE 4.1

Good Food Sources of Selenium

Food	Serving Size	Micrograms of Selenium per Serving
Bread		
White	1 slice	6.7
Whole wheat	1 slice	16.2
Eggs	1 large	12.0
Egg noodles	1 cup, cooked	105.0
Pasta	1 cup, cooked	90.0
Cereals		
Oats	1 ounce	12.6
Whole wheat	1 ounce	6.7
Rice (brown or white)	1 cup	21.6
Seafood (edible portion)		
Lobster tail	3½ ounces	63.4
Shrimp	3½ ounces	57.2
Cod, fillet	3½ ounces	46.5
Flounder, fillet	3½ ounces	33.5
Oyster	3½ ounces	64.6
Meat		
Beef, lean meat	3½ ounces	25.0
Pork, includes ham	3½ ounces	24.0
Vegetables		
Lima beans	½ cup	7.0
Most green vegetables	½ cup	3.0
Garlic, 3 cloves	⅓ ounce	2.5
Mushrooms, fresh	½ cup	4.3
Milk	8-ounce glass	14.3
Cheese, average	1 ounce	7.9
Chicken and turkey	3½ ounces	34.0

The values here are averaged from various sources including: *Journal of Food Science, ACTA Pharmacologica of Toxicologica* and *Bioinorganic Chemistry.*

Amounts of selenium in foods differ in most published sources; however, a person following the recommendations in the Longevity Diet should get over 75 micrograms of selenium daily.

The selenium content in food varies with the selenium content of the soil in which it's grown. The values shown on table 4.1 are averages for the United States. Food-producing regions in the United States and Canada have adequate soil selenium, so virtually all food (including livestock) will provide adequate selenium.

The following rules will help you get enough selenium:

- Eat a high-fiber cereal (wheat, oat, rice, corn) each day.

- Eat two servings daily of foods from whole grains, such as pasta or whole grain breads.

- Eat a clove of garlic or some onion each day, either cooked or raw.

- Eat fish three times weekly.

ARE SUPPLEMENTS OKAY? NECESSARY?

Selenium supplementation makes sense if protection is your aim. A daily multivitamin-mineral supplement containing 50 to 100 micrograms of selenium is definitely safe and healthy. The Longevity Diet will provide 50 to 75 micrograms daily of selenium from foods; say, an average of 60 micrograms. Therefore, an additional 50 to 150 micrograms of selenium in a supplement with a total of 200 to 250 micrograms is safely below a working upper limit of 300 micrograms and far below the mildly unsafe level of 1 milligram.

I follow the Longevity Diet and eat extra servings of selenium-rich foods, so I'm secure knowing I get about 60 micrograms of selenium daily. I also take a daily multivitamin-mineral supplement that provides 100 micrograms of selenium.

5

Taurine

In 1827, an unusual amino acid was found in the bile of the ox *Bos taurus*. The discoverers named it *taurine,* after taurus, the bull.

Taurine is unusual because unlike other amino acids, it's not used as a building block of protein; so we call it a "free" amino acid. For about one hundred and fifty years, scientists thought of it as nothing more than a component of bile.

Taurine Quiz

Answer yes or no to the following questions:

- If you are a mother, do or did you breastfeed your children?

- Are you a vegan-vegetarian (one who consumes no animal food or dairy products)?

- Do you consume a lot of alcoholic beverages?

- Have you or any blood relative had epilepsy, hepatitis, gallstones, or cystic fibrosis?

• Have you had trouble gaining weight due to fat malabsorption?

A yes to any of these questions should pique your curiosity about taurine. Being informed is a step to better health.

The liver produces bile acids, which are passed through the gall bladder to our digestive system, to digest and absorb fat. Bile acids are natural detergents that help us digest dietary fat much as household detergents make fat and grease dissolve off dishes into the dishwater. Since taurine is a component of bile, most scientists assumed it was just another natural emulsifier, so no one paid much attention to it. But in 1975, a paper appeared in the journal *Science* entitled "Retinal Degeneration Associated with Taurine Deficiency in the Cat." This paper reported that cats go blind when their diets are taurine deficient. Interesting, but "no cigar," unless cat breeding is your objective. Suspicions were raised as to taurine's role, however, and additional studies—some on humans—began.

Baby monkeys were raised on a taurine-deficient, human infant formula. Sure enough, they developed the same degeneration of the eye tissue seen in cats. Then, almost at the same time, research was published showing that some premature human infants developed similar symptoms.

In order to obtain the conditions necessary for these symptoms to occur in premature babies, they must have been kept alive by total parenteral nutrition, meaning that a tube is inserted into the baby's body through a vein and the infant is fed a mixture of the chemicals necessary for life; the child isn't fed milk. Taurine was left out of the mix because, at the time, it wasn't considered essential. However, since these scientific reports were published, taurine has been included in infant formulas under Pascal's philosophy that "it won't do any harm and there's evidence suggesting it does some good, so why not use it." Understandably, scientists cannot conduct research that would involve denying babies an essential nutrient, so the matter rests there for now.

Infants with an intestinal condition known as the blind-loop syndrome show the same tissue symptoms. As the name implies, a large part of the intestine is bypassed and nutrients aren't absorbed. In this case, the nutrient was coming from mother's milk. These observations confirmed that taurine isn't just a natural detergent as scientists thought but an important nutrient.

Anything in food that relates to the development of the visual tissues deserves a close look. Since the original paper was published in 1975 explaining that the ability of cats to see depends on taurine, more than twenty-six hundred scientific papers on taurine have appeared (by 1990), and research is still going strong.

Mother's milk is nature's most perfect food for infants. At childbirth, it consists of antibodies that kill bacteria in the infant's digestive system. Its iron is especially bound so that the baby can use the iron but not the germs, which also need the iron to grow. As the infant grows and his nutritional needs change, the composition of breast milk changes to satisfy those nutritional needs. Mother's milk continues to change as long as she nurses her baby.

At birth, the taurine level of mother's milk is at its highest. By five days, it has declined over 20 percent, and it declines even more after that. Since the fat in mother's milk increases after birth, you'd expect taurine amounts to also increase if it was there for fat digestion. A decline is the opposite of what you'd expect.

It didn't take scientists long after the 1975 paper on retina degeneration to prove that taurine isn't in mother's milk to digest fat. Indeed, experiments proved taurine made no difference in fat digestion or absorption for the infant. Obviously, it's there for another purpose. That purpose is development of the tissues required for vision and the function of several important glands.

Our body contains about 15 grams or about half an ounce of taurine. That makes us about 0.02 percent taurine by weight. Three fourths of this amount is in our muscles. The amount we lose each day varies according to how much we get in our diet and the quality of protein in our diet. The importance of taurine is more obvious if we look at its content in specific tissues.

Although we can get taurine directly from meat, our body makes most of the taurine we need. It is made from a sulfur-containing amino acid, cysteine, which we get from protein. Cysteine, an essential amino acid, is often found in only limited amounts in protein, so it is important that we get adequate amounts of high-quality protein. The best sources of cysteine are proteins of animal origin, including dairy products, but there are also some good vegetable sources, listed at the end of the chapter.

Taurine is most concentrated in the pineal and pituitary glands of the brain and the retina of the eye. Taurine concentration in the remainder of the brain is only exceeded by that of glutamic acid, which some brain cells use for energy. Among body muscles, the greatest concentration of taurine is in heart muscle. However, the larger amount of taurine is found in other muscles simply because they make up the bulk of body tissues.

The pituitary and pineal glands are located together in the brain. They produce many hormones that regulate growth, development, metabolism, water balance, and other bodily functions. If something goes wrong with either gland, the results can be disastrous. For example, a child can become a giant or midget and an adult can get diabetes. The importance of these glands to our health can't be overstated.

As an adult, your liver, brain, and other organs contain about half the concentration of taurine they did at birth. Similarly, a pregnant woman's placenta (or is it the infant's placenta?) contains more taurine than either the mother's or infant's liver. High concentrations of taurine in these tissues at birth illustrate a developmental need that declines with age, as the latter concentrations suggest. Nevertheless, its concentration in these same tissues in adults indicates that taurine has an important, ongoing role in health.

HOW DOES TAURINE WORK?

Taurine isn't a nutrient like a vitamin or dietary fiber. Its function in nerve and muscle tissue is more subtle and less precise than that of a vitamin: taurine keeps things in electrical balance, it prevents runaway nerve impulses. In terms of household electronics, you'd say it prevents power surges, a blown fuse or tripped circuit breaker.

Taurine's unique chemical structure means that in body tissues it's a "zwitterion." Zwitterion comes from German and means "middle ion." An ion is something with a charge, either positive or negative. "Middle" or "Zwitter" doesn't mean taurine has no charge; it means that it has the same amount of positive charge as negative charge, so "middle" or "zwitter" is a correct label. Taurine is neutral because it's both positive and negative.

Taurine's abundance in nervous system tissue, or in tissue, such as heart muscle, that has an important nerve function, is a clue to what it does. Taurine seems to balance electrical charges in these tissues and keep the currents flowing correctly. I use the word *currents* because nerves are the body's electrical wires and nerve impulses are measured as currents. Indeed, many modern medical devices rely on these impulses to collect their diagnostic information.

Unlike electrical wires in a house, which must be kept dry, nerves are bathed in body fluids and require an elaborate balance of electrical charges inside and outside to function properly. This charge balance does several things. Most importantly, the balance permits the nerve to transmit or ''fire'' a signal and be ready in a millisecond to fire again. If the charges around the nerves aren't correctly balanced, there can be unwanted firings of nerve impulses, or no firing at all. The result of this unbalance is chaos. For example, the brain won't function and the heart won't beat. This unbalance will cause death if it isn't corrected quickly.

Taurine's primary function seems to be balancing electrical charges in nervous system tissue, a supposition that explains its concentration in tissues intimately involved in nerve function: the brain, the eyes, heart muscle, and the pituitary and pineal glands.

No tissue is as sensitive to good nerve function as the eyes, and the retina is probably the most sensitive. Since cats don't make their own taurine, they must depend on their diet to provide it. Cats lose all ability to see when the retinal taurine level drops by 50 percent. If it drops more than 50 percent, the retina deteriorates physically and cats become permanently blind. Dietary taurine is obtained only from flesh; it's not surprising that cats of all sizes are carnivores. No other food source would work for them, so don't try to raise a vegetarian cat.

Since we can make our own taurine if our diet is correct, nature protects human eye and brain development in two ways: she makes sure there's plenty of taurine for the infant in the womb by concentrating it in the placenta and letting it cross into the infant; then she makes sure mother's milk supplies abundant amounts.

Now think about the high concentration of taurine in the pituitary and pineal glands, especially in infants. These tissues regulate the growth, development, and function of most organs. They depend critically on input of nerve impulses and hormone output. Their importance to the quality of human life can't be overstated. As is true in the case of the retina, it's essential that these glands develop within very precise guidelines and function properly, especially in the early years, for correct growth to occur.

Not surprisingly, the human brain continues to grow larger for up to eight years after birth. Deprive children of sufficient protein during this period and they will not develop correctly. Worse yet, they'll never fully recover even after adequate protein is restored. Since taurine is the most highly concentrated of all amino acids in the infant's brain, nature is saying, "Read my lips; taurine is important!"

Heart muscle is especially dependent on correct nerve and muscle fiber interaction. Electrical charge and impulses are critical not only in the nerves of the heart but also in its muscle fibers as well. If the impulses that make it work get mixed up, fibrillation occurs. Fibrillation is the random vibrating that is seen so commonly portrayed on TV dramas. On TV, it's usually straightened out by giving the heart a single, large electric shock with huge paddles held by a handsome paramedic. If the fibrillation is caused by not enough taurine, the paddles won't get it started again.

Taurine's role as a modulator of tissue function involves the regulation of electrical charge. This is most obvious in impulse conduction in nerves, but it has a place in other tissues as well. Cell membranes need to be stable because they regulate the amount of water, calcium, sodium, and potassium that goes in and out of each cell. And each cell requires just the right balance of calcium inside and outside. Taurine is essential in maintaining these balances, as well as water and ion balance. If the cell has an imbalance of water or ions or elements, it bursts or shrivels up from dehydration and dies. Taurine, with its unique balance of positive and negative charges, is ideally suited for the job. It acts as a type of "charge" reservoir. So, if you're a little short of calcium, which has a positive charge, or phosphate, which has a negative one, disaster won't occur, because taurine has both charges and can supply the charge that's needed. Even though the body can't make calcium or phosphorus, it can make taurine.

ANTIXENOBIOTICS

Taurine's role in tissue function is so important that its protective ability to neutralize dangerous toxins is usually overlooked. These toxins are produced within our own tissues and are correctly named xenobiotics. *Xeno*, from Greek, pronounced "zeno," means "strange," and *biotic* means "from living." So xenobiotics are strange chemicals produced within our own bodies.

Taurine reacts directly with two very critical xenobiotics. These xenobiotics are produced by the action of peroxide or active oxygen on chlorides and nitrates forming superoxides, dangerous materials that cause a breach of the cell membrane if they aren't neutralized. When the cell membrane is breached, other toxins can rush in and attack the genetic material. Taurine steps in and neutralizes some of these toxins by joining with them to form new nontoxic materials that eventually get excreted harmlessly in your urine.

If toxic superoxides aren't neutralized, they cause problems ranging from a serious breakdown of tissue function to cancer formation. So taurine performs other, protective functions in our blood and tissues besides modulating the electrical charge on nerve fibers and the electrical balance of cell membranes.

Retinoic acid can be made by the body from vitamin A and is important in the protection of skin from cancer. In fact, some scientists are searching for a link between retinoic acid and the prevention of some types of cancer. However, retinoic acid in some tissues is toxic. Excessive retinoic acid in pregnant women causes serious birth defects in their babies. So while retinoic acid is helpful in the skin and a few other tissues, it's a toxin in other tissues. In these other tissues, the retinoic acid is neutralized by taurine.

TAURINE IN THERAPY

Taurine is a protector that allows the correct development of critical tissues and a tissue protector against reactive xenobiotics. Does taurine have any therapeutic applications? Though our interest is in taurine's protective roles, insight for them is also gained and sharpened from therapy. We saw in chapter 3 that the therapeutic effects of beta carotene on skin pigment diseases helped us understand its protective function.

This is a listing of investigations being done now in which taurine is suspected of having or is known to have a therapeutic effect.

- *Cardiovascular disease:* Positive results have been documented in cases of congestive heart failure. Some cases have been classified as the result of taurine deficiency.

- *Cystic fibrosis steatorrhea:* A condition that results from a patient's inability to absorb fat. Taurine has a positive therapeutic effect—it reduces symptoms of fat malabsorption.

- *Gallstone treatment:* Supplemental taurine helps remove residual cholesterol and reduce gallstone formation.

- *Liver disorders in hepatitis:* Taurine has been effective in reducing symptoms of liver failure and speeding recovery.

- *Myotonic dystrophy:* An inherited disorder in which muscles contract correctly but don't relax, characterized by a reduced life span and serious complications. Taurine produces significant improvement.

These illnesses are suspected of having some aspects of a taurine dysfunction. By dysfunction, I mean that people have these illnesses because they may need more taurine than normal, because they excrete too much in their urine, because their liver doesn't make enough, or because they don't reabsorb it from their intestines.

ALCOHOLISM

Alcohol causes excessive taurine excretion. So, in advanced alcoholism, you'd expect problems associated with taurine depletion. A reasonable expectation would be that alcohol-related dementia is a result of the lowered taurine concentration in the brain. If the dementia was taurine-related, you'd expect supplemental taurine to reduce the episodes and help stabilize recovery.

Taurine was given to severe, randomly selected alcoholics entering withdrawal, and they were compared to similarly severe alcoholics in withdrawal who didn't get taurine. Of the taurine-treated alcoholics, only 14 percent had psychotic episodes compared to 45 percent of the nontaurine treated. In a more selective study, only psychotic alcoholics were selected. In psychotic alcoholics compared after admission to treatment, taurine reduced the episodes from 64 percent to 6 percent; in short, it reduced them by 90 percent! A 90-percent reduction says clearly that taurine is helping stabilize a mental condition.

EPILEPSY

Epilepsy is a disease in which the nerve cells in the brain don't function correctly. It is characterized by seizures, uncontrolled motor activity, altered consciousness, and inappropriate behavior. It's as if the brain goes out of control and has no modulator to keep nerve impulses in order. In the early 1970s, a few specialists gave epileptics large amounts of taurine in their search for a way to slow this terrible disease. This early 1970s research couldn't be built on animal studies, because epilepsy doesn't develop in animals; therefore, these early experiments were a form of high-level trial-and-error clinical research, with subjects being chosen at random and dosages initiated arbitrarily.

These studies were not double-blind as is preferred in medical research, so their findings are open to question. In spite of their design, all these trials produced positive results that varied from 16- to 90-percent seizure reduction. The level of seizure reduction depended on subjective conclusions about seizure reduction. If you accept the low-end results of 16-percent reduction as valid, there's no doubt that an outstanding effect was observed. Sixteen-percent reduction is important enough to warrant continued research, but clinicians need to select test cases of epilepsy more carefully, as was done on the test with alcoholics.

A careful review of the test cases suggests that the bodies of some epileptics don't handle taurine normally. Their intracellular levels of taurine are lower than normal because their excretion rate is much higher than normal. Consequently, they are likely to be helped by supplemental taurine. In contrast, other patients' bodies handle taurine normally, so their epileptic seizures are not caused by inadequate taurine; it's something else. Future studies will probably indicate that some epileptics are helped with taurine, while others aren't. Indeed, it's even possible that we will find some epileptics are partially taurine deficient and can be cured very easily.

TAURINE IN BILE

Bile acids are important for the emulsification of fat. They're produced in the liver, passed into the gall bladder, and passed out through the bile duct into the intestine. The removal of bile acids from the body by fiber helps reduce their reabsorption and indirectly lowers cholesterol. Taurine has an important effect on bile acids, as well.

Bile acids combine with taurine to form complex materials called taurine conjugates, which are essential for fat utilization. They also help to mobilize cholesterol and reduce gallstone formation. This could be interpreted as a detoxification by taurine. Since some bile acids are toxic, their reaction with taurine neutralizes the toxicity. In this context, bile acids are toxic and taurine is a protector.

WHERE DO WE GET TAURINE?

Once past infancy, you can normally make sufficient taurine if you get dietary protein of good quality and in sufficient quantity. If you eat meat or fish, you'll also get taurine directly. So if you're not a strict vegetarian, you'll get adequate dietary taurine or make all you require.

If you follow the Longevity Diet, your diet will contain from 200 to 400 milligrams of taurine daily. This is an effective level. Additionally, your diet will contain protein of sufficient quantity and quality so that your body can make enough taurine even if your dietary supply runs short.

VEGAN-VEGETARIANS

Vegan-vegetarians—who avoid all animal products—run a modest risk of not getting enough good-quality protein. This puts them at risk of not getting enough sulfur-containing amino acids to make their taurine. This deficiency can be overcome by eating a broad variety of foods, with an emphasis on beans, mushrooms, and rice.

SAFETY

Taurine is concentrated in many tissues at concentrations four hundred to six hundred times the amount in blood. This indicates that it is safe at high dietary levels and there is no known toxicity.

SOURCES OF TAURINE

Foods with Taurine

- Meat and poultry
- Fish and shellfish

Foods with Sulfur-containing Amino Acids (From Highest to Lowest)

- Milk and dairy products
- Soybean flour and soy protein
- Nuts
- Beans
- Pasta
- Mushrooms
- Tofu

P A R T

II

REGULATORS

Your body is constantly growing. Some cells divide every fourteen days; others every eight weeks. In the time it takes to read this paragraph, your body has made one hundred thousand new red blood cells and has gotten rid of one hundred thousand old ones. Did you ever wonder how your body keeps everything going in the right direction?

Say one cell division in ten million goes wrong; then say one of those in ten million is cancerous. That yields about one hundred and eighty-five chances of getting cancer by age fifty. This calculation only considers random mistakes and doesn't count the assaults on our cells from the noxious materials in food, water, or the air. With all the other causes of mistakes, you might ask, "How come there's not more cancer?"

More mistakes in cell division don't show up because there is a network of systems to correct these mistakes when they are made and materials—such as antioxidant protectors—to prevent them from happening in the first place. We call this safety network redundant because there are usually two systems that correct each possible error. Since life has been on earth for about four billion years and man for over three million years, it's reasonable to expect that some reliable methods of prevention have developed.

REGULATOR PROTECTORS

Each body function, from those involving the simplest biochemical reaction to entire tissues and organs, is regulated by various biochemical mechanisms. Regulation often depends on dietary components I call regulatory protectors, which influence the direction and tone of entire body systems. In contrast to hormones, which our body produces in minute amounts to regulate body functions, we get the regulatory protectors from food. If the protectors aren't present in sufficient quantity or the right balance at the appropriate time, entire systems won't work or develop as they should. The accumulative effect of inadequate amounts of these regulatory protectors is severely debilitating, if not completely disastrous.

Some protectors, like the essential oils, are ingredients in the regulatory process, and the balance between the omega-3 and omega-6 oils is important. Other regulatory protectors, like folic acid, are similar to tools in the developmental process and remain after the job is done. Your body trying to manage without folic acid is like a mechanic working without the right parts; the job just doesn't come out right, if it can get done at all.

Your body is the pinnacle of life as we know it. Each of its fifty trillion cells live in a harmonious relationship with one another. All that's required of us is to provide the cells and tissues with the proper nutrients in good balance so all our systems have the basic substance to work correctly. We can get adequate regulatory protectors by developing a few good food habits.

Fiber

Many modern health problems are in part due to the decline in the amount of fiber we eat. This decline parallels the increase in industrialization but has accelerated in recent decades with the proliferation of processed foods and convenience eating. Since we live longer now and because fiber effects accumulate slowly, the results of inadequate fiber have more time to develop, as they tend to show up as we get older. This makes fiber deficiency harmful because its results don't emerge until it's too late to apply correct dietary measures. Indeed, fiber proves that prevention is the best medicine.

Fiber Quiz

These questions deal with one of the most important protectors of your health. Answer the questions with a yes or no:

- Are you irregular in your bowel movements, i.e., you don't have a bowel movement with firm, light brown stools once every twenty-four to thirty-six hours?

- Have you or a blood relative ever had gallstones or gall bladder disease?

- Have you or a blood relative ever had diverticulosis, hemorrhoids, appendicitis, or varicose veins in the thighs?

- If you're over the age of thirty-five, is your total cholesterol less than 200 milligrams per deciliter of blood? Is your HDL cholesterol over 50 milligrams per deciliter?

- Have you or any blood relative ever had cancer of the colon or rectum, or polyps?

A yes answer to any of these questions means that chapters 6 and 7 could have a profound effect on your health. More, if you apply the knowledge you gain, you could increase the quality and quantity of your life.

WHAT IS DIETARY FIBER?

Dietary fiber is the indigestible part of plant foods. It passes through the stomach and small intestine without being digested. Digestion of food begins in the mouth with chewing, accelerates in the stomach with acid and digestive enzymes, and is completed by enzymes in the thirteen or more feet of the small intestine. In the large intestine, more digestion takes place as fermentation.

In contrast to active digestion in the small intestine, microbial digestion or fermentation is accomplished by the microbes that inhabit the large intestine. These microbes convert some fiber and undigested food fractions to other substances. No fiber is digested in the small intestine, but some fiber is fermented in the large intestine. Consequently, the definition of dietary fiber means it's not digested by human digestive juices even though our normal bacteria can digest some fiber.

Next time you walk through a supermarket, drive by a farm, read a menu, or glance through a magazine, notice the incredible variety of fruits, vegetables, and edible flowers. I'm not sure anyone knows how many plant foods there are, because besides the major varieties like wheat, apples, beans, and spinach, there are varieties within each group like red and bulgar wheat, delicious and macintosh apples, or kidney and pinto beans. Then there are the obscure varieties. The important thing to remember is that each one of them provides its own unique dietary fiber.

When we process foods we change their fiber, so in addition to the unique fiber each plant food contains, there are myriad man-made fiber product variations, such as wheat, oat, rice, apple, and corn to name an obvious few. We'll return to the issue of variation, but now let's look at the basic functions of fiber.

When you get enough correctly balanced fiber, it works for you in two ways. It prevents watery or hard stools and produces firm, but soft, easily moved stools. When you're getting the right amount and right mix of fiber, you'll move light brown stools once in twenty-four to thirty-six hours. That's why I call fiber ''nature's regulator.'' To regulate your body correctly, you have to get enough fiber in the correct proportions and drink enough water, because without water fiber is similar to sawdust or even a kind of glue, depending on its source.

How much fiber is enough? Extensive research has proven that to have stools every twenty-four to thirty-six hours requires about twenty-five to forty grams of fiber daily. About two-thirds should be hard or insoluble fiber and the other third soft or soluble fiber. The next chapter translates this one ounce of fiber into foods you eat regularly.

Plant cell walls are a matrix of six types of fiber depending on where the plant grows and how it propagates itself. For example, a wheat grain has an outer coat that's tough and hard to withstand the elements and keep the contents of the grain intact. The fiber in this outer coat is bran or hard fiber. Bran is mostly cellulose and could probably be made into paper like this page, if necessary, although trees provide a better source of the cellulose used for paper.

In another example, grains of corn are protected inside a husk and are supported on a cob. The corn husk protects its contents sufficiently for the reproduction of the corn plant, so the outer layer of a corn kernel is softer than wheat is.

An apple has a different fiber matrix. The skin is obviously tough: It keeps the apple from drying out and provides resistance to insects. But it's soft enough so the ripe fruit can be easily eaten by animals and man. In contrast, the matrix of the apple seed is tougher than that of the wheat grain, allowing it to pass through the digestive systems of animals, birds, and man unharmed. This toughness allows the seed to be transported long distances by animals and birds and passed in their stools. The seed coat can then be broken by freezing or scraping so the seed can swell with water, germinate, and a new tree can grow.

Insoluble fiber is hard and generally resistant to digestion by most animals and microorganisms and to fermentation by microbes in our intestinal tract. Supermarket sources of insoluble fiber are usually cereals and have the word *bran* in the title. Thus wheat bran, oat bran, corn bran, rice bran, and even unprocessed bran are all sources of insoluble fiber. High-fiber cereals usually contain some insoluble fiber, often from wheat. Insoluble fiber is mostly cellulose; all vegetable foods contain some insoluble fiber. Grains and cereals are, without question, the best sources. Insoluble hard fiber swells in water but doesn't dissolve in it.

All plants contain varying amounts of soft or soluble fiber. It helps to create the fiber matrix and holds the plant cells together. A good example are the gums in oatmeal, beans, and some vegetables. *Gum's* a good term.

As is true in all natural materials, there are many gradations between the two fiber extremes; most plants contain some of all of them, even though one type of fiber might dominate. We have identified six general types of dietary fiber with hard, insoluble bran at one extreme and gums at the other. Although fiber exists to help the plant stand tall, making it possible to reach sunlight and better able to reproduce, we've adapted to the availability and functions of each type of fiber. We depend on fiber just as we rely on vitamins. However, the body functions that call for fiber are far more subtle than those that require vitamins, so our dependence on fiber isn't as obvious as it is on vitamins.

TABLE 6.1

The Six Types of Fiber

	Water Soluble	Function in Plant	Food Sources
Cellulose	No	Forms structure of cell walls with lignins	Wheat bran, fruit peels, seed coats
Lignin	No	Forms structure of cell walls with cellulose	Cereal grains, potato skins

Hemicellulose	Partly	Holds cells together with cellulose	Wheat bran, grains
Pectin	Yes	Binds cells together and holds water in fruit	Fruits
Gum	Yes	Binds stems, seeds, and vegetables	Oatmeal, legumes, vegetables
Mucilages	Yes	Binds in seeds; binds stems in aquatic plants	Seaweed, seeds

A vitamin deficiency produces a well-defined set of symptoms in a month or so. Restore the vitamin and the symptoms start to disappear in a few days. In contrast, a fiber deficiency may start in childhood and show up as diverticulosis or hemorrhoids at age forty. By then, the cause of the illness is too remote to be relevant. Taking fiber when you have diverticulosis can relieve the symptoms but can't reverse the damage that has been done. This is a good time to get back to the story of the lack of fiber as a deficiency disease.

LOW FIBER VERSUS HIGH FIBER

Food contains three major classes of nutrients—proteins, fats, and carbohydrates. Food also provides water and, within the carbohydrates, fiber. Daily, we eat about one pound in dry weight of food. That means that if you took a day's worth of food and removed all the water, it would weigh about a pound. So if you increase one component of the food, you've got to decrease another if you're going to stay within the same one pound of dry weight. For example, a high-fat diet will be low in carbohydrates because foods that are high in fat are usually low in carbohydrates. Since fat is usually found in animal food, a high-fat diet is likely to be a high-protein diet, as well. However, if your diet consisted largely of fish, grains, and vegetables, it would be a high-protein, high-carbohydrate, low-fat diet, because fish is an animal protein generally low in fat.

Because we generally eat enough food to satisfy our energy or calorie needs, and because fat supplies more than twice the energy as the same amount of carbohydrates, a high-fat diet will weigh less than a high-carbohydrate diet providing the same number of calories. However, since we eat about a pound of dry weight, the person on a high-fat diet tends to weigh more, because there are more calories in high-fat foods.

A high-carbohydrate diet is a bulky diet. Fiber and carbohydrates bind water and make it bulky. You can see this by comparing a piece of chocolate to an apple.

A one-ounce square of milk chocolate supplies about 150 calories; just about twice what you get from a medium apple at 80 calories. You can swallow the chocolate in a gulp, but the apple takes some chewing. The chocolate is 1 percent water; fat and sugar don't hold water. The apple is 84 percent water! The water in the apple is bound to the carbohydrates, especially the fiber, which includes pectin and cellulose. Since experts say our need to chew is basic, a high-carbohydrate diet takes more space, satisfies our chewing need with greater bulk while it supplies fewer calories pound for pound. You eat more and feel fuller with fewer calories.

DENNIS BURKITT, THE FIBER MAN

Dennis Burkitt, a deeply religious Irishman, decided to study medicine at Trinity College by chance. Like many students, he didn't know what to select as his major, so he wrote initials representing his options on scraps of paper, shuffled them in a box, blindfolded himself, and pulled one out. Fortunately for us, he got an "M" (for medicine).

Dr. Burkitt had two unusual habits: he made a practice of getting to know his patients, and, when possible, he participated in their religious meetings. He also kept a daily diary summarizing his observations on each patient's needs and problems. These habits, married to his keen insight, helped him to cut through complex medical problems with clear simplicity. His insights have a remarkable clarity.

Posted to Africa in 1944 during World War II, he stayed on as a medical missionary. An unusually gifted physician, he had identified the cause and developed the preventive method for an infectious disease of the testicles. More importantly, he had characterized an unusual form of cancer, named Burkitt's lymphoma after his monumental work on it.

Burkitt's lymphoma is an unusual cancer that affects children. Burkitt had found its cause, cure, and even preventive approaches. His work on this terrible cancer is a milestone of modern medicine.

A MODERN DEFICIENCY DISEASE

In 1960, Dr. Hugh Trowell, a medical missionary in Africa and a friend of Burkitt's, published his book entitled *Noninfectious Diseases in Africa*. He presented the startling hypothesis that most noninfectious diseases of the digestive tract were really deficiency diseases, caused by a lack of something in the diet. Trowell included diverticulosis, hemorrhoids, colon cancer, and colitis, among others, in this grouping. He claimed they were caused by a deficiency of unrefined carbohydrates—starches and fiber.

When Trowell's book came out in 1960, Burkitt was intrigued. He decided to see for himself if his friend was correct. He used his diary with its personal knowledge of his patients to forge his own conclusions.

Burkitt noticed a distinct difference in the noninfectious digestive diseases between the native Africans and English people working in Africa. He saw similar distinctions between Africans and Englishmen living in the cities and those living in the country. These disparities convinced him that color or ethnic origins weren't the difference.

Burkitt observed that the South African city dwellers ate a low-fiber, high-fat diet typical of people living in England. He observed that the country folks ate a low-fat, high-fiber diet more typical of the natives. He also observed the stools of both groups. In the country, stools were soft, light brown, large, and moved daily. In the city, stools were hard, dark, small, and moved once in three to five days.

Burkitt's diary took him much further than how often people moved their bowels. He could compare their illnesses to the frequency of bowel movements and dietary fiber. His observations were startling at the time. They are even more startling today, since they have been confirmed by more modern research methods. I've summarized these observations, as revised by more recent findings, in table 6.2.

TABLE 6.2

Noninfective Bowel Diseases
in South African Populations

	Rural Blacks (never urban)	Urban Blacks (raised in rural)	Urban Whites (always urban)
Dietary fiber, grams per day	40 or more	25 or more	17 or less

FIBER-RELATED ILLNESSES

Hemorrhoids	Rare	+ +	+ + +
Appendicitis	+	+ +	+ + + + +
Ulcerative colitis	Rare	+	+ + + + +
Irritable bowel syndrome	+	+ +	+ + + +
Diverticular disease	Rare	+	+ + + + +
Colon cancer	Rare	+	+ + + + +

The rate at which an illness appears is indicated by the symbol +, with + being the illness seen occasionally and + + + + + being the illness as a serious cause of death or debilitation.

These data are taken from many research papers. For a review, see: "Epidemiology of Noninfective Bowel Diseases in South African Populations," A. R. P. Walker and I. Segal, *Tropical Gastroenterology* 4:155 (1983).

Burkitt concluded from these observations that a refined diet didn't provide enough fiber. In addition, he called the illnesses this lack of fiber generated "deficiency diseases." He published this work in 1965.

How did people respond to Burkitt's hypothesis? They didn't! Nothing happened! Scientists are busy with their own projects. Consequently, when a new concept is published, it doesn't get a lot of attention; that takes time. I read Burkitt's papers and decided to publish one in the United States. In 1972 I submitted a paper entitled "Fiber, the Forgotten Nutrient" to a scientific journal. After some debate, they published the paper in early 1973. The referees said, "It's a fine example for students of how a paper should be written, but the subject is unimportant." This paper has been cited and reproduced many times. It proves that seven years after Burkitt's book on fiber, experts still thought the subject was unimportant.

GETTING ATTENTION: A BURKITT SEMINAR

Dennis Burkitt, an unusually gifted speaker, had a new mission in life: to make people aware of the need for fiber. His loud, clear voice captured the audience's attention, while his humorous approach told his story. His presentations generally went something like this.

* Slide one was a cartoon of an overflowing sink with people in white coats frantically mopping up the floor. The overflowing sink represented illness, while the people mopping the floor characterized physicians treating symptoms. Going for the cure meant turning off the faucet and unclogging the drain—dealing with the cause.
* Slides two through five were stools. Big, soft, light brown plops from country dwellers and small, dark brown, oily stools of city dwellers. Imagine the embarrassment of people attending the seminar. Many people don't talk about this subject, let alone look at it on the "big screen." After sweating through these slides, though, you certainly knew what type of stools were good for you.
* Slides six through ten were toilets. English toilets like thrones. American hotel rooms with telephones by the toilet. He would compare these toilets to the low toilets of the Orient or Middle East (no telephones with these). This was a shock treatment introduction to toilet rituals and a comparison that said low toilets are best.

After the slide presentation and narrative, Burkitt would show data to prove that many modern intestinal disorders are really fiber-deficiency diseases.

FIBER-DEFICIENCY DISEASES IN BURKITT'S HYPOTHESIS

Burkitt's 1965 insights have been verified by other scientists, who with more research have added other illnesses to the list. Most of Burkitt's hypotheses are valid today, so I use his words to explain them, although cancer is far more complex than he thought in 1965.

Diseases that Dennis Burkitt identified as fiber-deficiency diseases are summarized on table 6.2, revised and upgraded to 1990 standards.

Hemorrhoids

Painful hemorrhoids develop when veins in the rectum, near the anus, become inflamed. When inflamed, these veins extend outside the opening of the anus, and they hurt. Burkitt reasoned that hemorrhoids start to develop at a young age from the pressure people on a low-fiber diet must exert to pass their stools. Toilet height is another story. He'd explain how the Englishman had to ''push'' while sitting on a high, thronelike toilet to get his stools out. While you're sitting and pushing, the blood in the veins lining the anus doesn't flow back toward the heart very well; it ''pools'' in the veins, and they swell. As Burkitt said: ''Do that for forty years, the veins weaken, and you have hemorrhoids.'' When the inflammation doesn't subside, or hemorrhoids recur frequently or burst, surgical removal is the only solution.

Appendicitis

A small pouch about two inches long runs off the large intestine where it connects with the small intestine. The pouch serves no modern purpose today that scientists can detect, so *appendix* is a good name. Biologists think that tens of thousands of years ago the appendix served as a fermentation pouch, a sort of extra stomach in which microbes could digest grains and other tough materials to get extra nourishment from vegetable foods. Since man didn't develop in a land of abundant food, this hypothesis seems likely.

Experience taught Burkitt that appendicitis is a Western dietary problem, and he reasoned that it had to do with our lack of fiber. Consequently, he theorized that appendicitis develops when food moves too slowly through our intestinal tract from a lack of fiber. He reasoned that in slow stool movement, pressure builds and forces the stool into the appendix. Since he presented this idea, researchers have proved that pressure inside your intestine is many times higher if you're on a low-fiber than on a high-fiber diet, indirectly confirming Burkitt's hypothesis. Pressure builds when the normal squeezing motion, called *peristalsis,* used to move the intestinal contents along encounters the resistance from hard stool.

Burkitt further reasoned that some undigested material gets forced into the appendix under high internal pressure. Once inside the appendix, undigested food materials can't exit if the pressure is too high because the valve to the small intestine closes it off from the large intestine. The appendix then acts like a pouch in which natural microbes ferment the appendix contents. Fermentation produces some irritating byproducts that cause swelling and close the appendix opening. The appendix is now infected and, if it isn't removed, it can burst. When it bursts, microorganisms spread throughout the abdomen, spreading infection. A burst appendix was sure death in the 1930s. It's still a serious problem today, even with antibiotics.

DIVERTICULOSIS

In 1965, diverticulosis was called a degenerative disease of aging; the idea was we would all get it if we lived long enough. As the large intestine ages along with the rest of us, small pouches or weak points develop in the spaces between the muscle bands that encircle it. Think of the large intestine as a long, flexible tube with muscles wrapped around it like string continuously wrapped around a bent hose. Now visualize the weak points developing between the string—muscle fibers—that wrap around the bends. If the internal pressure gets high enough wherever there's a weak point, a small bubble can form in the intestinal wall between the muscle bands. This bubblelike pouch is more correctly called a *diverticula.* Hence the name *diverticulosis,* meaning many pouches. On an X ray they actually look like little balloons along the intestinal wall.

It hurts just to think of stools or gas from stools filling these little pouches. When they become filled and inflamed, they're painful. If the pouch becomes too inflamed, it can burst. In its active form, the disease is called *diverticulitis*. When the diverticula are filled, bacteria in the stools continue fermenting, producing gas and irritating toxic materials. Surgical removal of the inflicted part of the intestine was the most common course when Burkitt wrote his papers in the 1960s.

Burkitt proposed that a high-fiber diet would not only prevent diverticulosis, but also relieve the symptoms even after the disease was established. Although this hypothesis was proposed by a few physicians in the 1930s, no one had paid attention. No physician had ever spoken so loudly, or with as much authority, as Dennis Burkitt.

Neil Painter, a quiet surgeon at the Manor House Hospital in London, heard Burkitt speak several times. The visions of people straining stuck in his mind. He believed Burkitt's hypothesis, so he offered his patients with diverticulosis the opportunity to test Burkitt's approach. I retraced his experiment with him in 1973, so I'll recall the story in his words as my notes indicate:

"I heard Dr. Burkitt speak. He was captivating! I decided to test his ideas on patients who wanted to try. The next day I stopped at the health food store and purchased some unprocessed wheat bran. I gave each volunteer patient with painful diverticulosis a large tablespoon and a bag of wheat bran. I instructed them to eat a spoonful of bran three times a day with meals."

His first attempt included seventy-two patients whose diverticulosis was bad enough to call for surgery. After using the bran, only seven ever required surgery to this day! The others remained in fine health as long as they kept using bran. The rest is history. Painter published his results in the *British Medical Journal.*

Subsequent, more sophisticated studies than Painter's proved that 90 percent of diverticulosis could be stopped with bran. In spite of better statistics and more sophisticated methods of diagnosis, the bottom line is clear: dietary fiber relieves the symptoms of diverticulosis! Painter proved that Burkitt was correct. Later studies show that it's best for people with diverticulosis to build their bran intake slowly, not all at once, as Painter's patients did. This advice is correct for anyone who hasn't had sufficient fiber. Start slowly and build. We'll go into this more in chapter 7.

DIVERTICULOSIS IN THE 1990s

In the twenty-five years since Burkitt first described diverticulosis as a deficiency disease, the epidemic has become worse. In 1965, experts called it a disease of aging. In those days, a specialist who looked hard enough could find some diverticulosis in about 60 percent of patients over the age of fifty. The actual number increases with age, which is consistent with a degenerative disease.

In 1990, diverticulosis appears more frequently in people under the age of fifty than in 1965, and now even appears in people under the age of thirty. It's no longer correct to call it a disease of aging since young people get it. The disease probably takes as much time to develop, but people don't get enough fiber starting at an increasingly early age, and some develop it more easily than others. This decline in age of onset proves some change in our diet speeds development of diverticulosis. We don't eat enough fiber. It's that simple.

In 1900, people consumed about thirty grams of fiber, about an ounce, daily; the amount most experts agree is basic to good health. We consumed twelve grams, on average, in 1990! For example, the typical diet provides just under six grams per 1000 calories. Since most women get along nicely on less than 2000 calories and most men on less than 2,500, a little arithmetic tells you that we get less than half of the fiber we need.

A PERSONAL EXPERIENCE WITH DIVERTICULOSIS

In 1978, five years after my paper entitled ''Fiber, the Forgotten Nutrient'' appeared, I was a speaker at a meeting of the Society of Food Technologists. After my talk, a man came up to me and asked to shake my hand. I asked why as we shook. He explained how, in 1973, he had been hospitalized for diverticulosis and was going to have surgery. He brought the journal with my paper for reading the night before surgery.

He showed my paper to his surgeon and asked if he could test a high-fiber diet for a while. The surgeon said, ''Sure, surgery can always be done.'' The man never did have surgery. Simply eating All-Bran cereal worked for him. I never told him the journal referees said the subject was unimportant.

HEART DISEASE

Burkitt claimed that heart disease indirectly involves fiber deficiency. By itself, a high-fiber diet is a low-fat, low-sugar diet because foods high in fiber are naturally low in fats and sugars. That's important, because fat and sugar cause heart disease. Burkitt went a step further and said that fiber reduces blood cholesterol. Blood cholesterol is the major indicator of heart disease, and all experts agree that keeping the level of blood cholesterol down is important in preventing heart disease. The blood cholesterol/heart disease relationship is widely accepted by experts.

Fiber reduces cholesterol in two ways. First, it directly binds dietary cholesterol, thus allowing it to pass out through the stools. Second, and more important, fiber binds bile acids and eliminates them. Once you understand how bile-acid elimination works, you'll see why Burkitt was correct when he suggested fiber could prevent gallstones.

Your liver makes 85 percent of the cholesterol in your body. Some cholesterol is converted to bile acids, which pass from the gall bladder into the intestine through the bile duct. Bile acids are necessary for good digestion. In the absence of fiber, these bile acids get absorbed further down the intestinal tract and returned to the liver for reuse. Absorption and reuse of bile acids reduce the need to convert more cholesterol into more bile acids; therefore, cholesterol is passed into the blood or, in some cases, even passed into the intestine. When adequate fiber is available, it binds bile acids—preventing their reuse—and so they're eliminated. It's like eliminating cholesterol, because your body then must break down more cholesterol to form more bile acids.

There's more, though, because a low-fiber diet is naturally high in fat and sugar. Fat goes indirectly into the blood via the lymphatic system (a secondary circulatory system that transports fat, as veins and arteries transport blood). However, in the absence of fiber, sugar goes directly into the blood and by raising your blood sugar level abruptly causes the body to think "extra calories," even if they aren't extra. An intake of sugar without fiber also causes the body to raise blood fat. Cholesterol is then necessary to stabilize the extra blood fat, so the liver makes more cholesterol. So a high-fiber, low-fat diet lowers cholesterol in two ways.

Cholesterol is a waxy substance that becomes the major component of plaque that causes clogged arteries that lead to heart disease. The more cholesterol we have in our blood, the greater the clogging of our arteries, and, conversely, the lower the cholesterol level is in our blood, the clearer our arteries. So the objective is to keep cholesterol as low as possible. Indeed, in 1988, the surgeon general set a target level of 200 milligrams or less for blood cholesterol. An eating pattern of high-fiber, low-fat foods will naturally produce low blood-cholesterol levels.

GALLSTONES

Burkitt's diary also showed that people who eat high-fiber foods didn't have gallstones. The bile duct passes bile into the small intestine. Bile is a greenish fluid that contains bile acids and cholesterol. Bile also contains materials that are byproducts of liver metabolism. Fiber also helps to remove them.

Cholesterol is necessary to stabilize fat for absorption in the intestine, as it does in the blood, so it's produced in the liver and passed in via the bile duct. People who eat lots of fat need more cholesterol in their intestines as well as in their blood. When the cholesterol in the bile duct gets too high, it forms a small cholesterol crystal. On a continued high-fat diet, the crystal continues to grow into a good-sized stone. Gallstones can get as large as golf balls. When people get lots of fiber, their diet is naturally low in fat, so the bile isn't full of cholesterol. And the level of self-made cholesterol remains low because fiber is binding bile acids and preventing their reuse, so your body must break down more cholesterol to produce more bile acids. A stone never forms because the cholesterol level remains low.

Sometimes stones form in the bile duct or gall bladder and cause a blockage, a process called gall bladder disease. Gallstones must be removed either by surgery or by being broken into small pieces by sound waves and eliminated naturally. Gallstones are almost pure cholesterol. They form in the gall bladder or bile duct because there's more cholesterol than can be dissolved in the bile.

INFLAMMATORY BOWEL DISEASES

A number of inflammatory intestinal disorders were observed by Burkitt that seem to be related to the amount of dietary fiber we eat. These include colitis, ulcerative colitis, and irritable bowel syndrome. His hypothesis is that insufficient fiber helped initiate these diseases through irritation.

There may be a weakness in your digestive system—perhaps in your muscles or in the lining of the intestines. If you don't get enough dietary fiber, that weakness will be under stress from the higher-than-normal pressure necessary for peristalsis to move the digested food through your whole system. Enough stress in the presence of other, complicating factors can result in physical damage. Once these diseases are established, it's too late. Adding fiber to your diet won't relieve the symptoms. Fiber can't restore the intestine to normal anymore than it can restore a heart damaged by poor diet and neglect.

Indeed, Burkitt seems to be correct in his theory that lack of fiber plays a role in the development of these diseases. However, heredity, stress, and the omega-3 oils discussed in chapter 8 are also involved in the onset of these diseases. Unfortunately, the development of these diseases involves the immune system, so once established, they're very complex.

CANCER

Burkitt's hypothesis stated and research confirmed that material moves through the intestinal tract more quickly in the presence of fiber. It follows then that when you eat a high-fiber diet, toxic materials should spend less time in the intestines before they're eliminated in the stools. In addition, a high-fiber diet produces stools that are about 75 percent water, so toxins are dissolved in the stool matrix more effectively. Armed with this simple reasoning, Burkitt observed the differences in intestinal cancer shown on table 6.2. Low fiber equates to high levels of colorectal cancer.

Since 1965, scientists have shown that diet and colonic cancer are interconnected. They've examined rates of colonic cancer in different countries and among different people. They've examined the rates of colonic cancer in men and women who have emigrated to our country and left a brother or sister in the old country. The results are the same. Shift from low-fat, high-fiber, high-carbohydrate foods to high-fat, low-fiber, low-carbohydrate foods, and the risk of intestinal cancer increases.

BEN ERSHOFF: ANIMAL STUDIES

Dr. Ben Ershoff, a scientist at the University of Southern California, proved that Burkitt was correct in his hypothesis that fiber detoxified some toxins. The same studies proved that fiber is a complex nutrient.

Ershoff did simple experiments. He put some rats on a basic diet and added a toxic material until they hardly grew and showed signs of dying; then he added fiber to the toxic diet. His reasoning was that, if Burkitt was correct, the fiber would bind up and neutralize the toxins. He confirmed Burkitt's hypothesis in animal studies.

Dr. Ershoff would make normal animal chow toxic by adding an excess amount of some toxic material—an artificial color, an industrial detergent, or even an artificial sweetener. Typically, he would reduce growth to 20 percent of normal with only 20 percent of the animals surviving. He would then repeat the experiment with various sources of fiber added to the food. The results were consistent. Some types of fiber, such as from alfalfa, would restore growth completely to normal. Other types of fiber such as wheat bran would partially restore growth, and some, such as purified cellulose, had very little effect.

By these studies, Dr. Ershoff not only proved that fiber would make a toxic diet safe, but also proved that some fiber worked better than others. He found that soluble fiber was most detoxifying. So, he proved that fiber sources such as alfalfa and psyllium, which are sources of soluble fiber, are better for detoxification than wheat bran, which is strictly hard, insoluble fiber, and produces regularity.

POLYPS AND COLORECTAL CANCER

Cancer of the large intestine, colon, and rectum (colorectal cancer) is like most other cancers; it starts slowly as a few dysplastic cells (see ''Bloody Mary,'' in chapter 1). One or more small, noncancerous growths, called polyps, develop somewhere in the colon or rectum. A polyp looks like a small bump when it starts and matures into a small protrusion, somewhat like a wart or a mole. More polyps develop as you get older; about one-third of all people over the age of fifty will have a few polyps somewhere in their large intestine.

Polyps are also found more frequently in people who have chronic constipation. Regularity again! A polyp is a clump of dysplastic cells, and some are more like cancer cells than normal cells. When polyps were found in former President Ronald Reagan during a routine physical, they were removed the very next day. Doctors don't take chances with a president!

Polyps are the prelude to intestinal cancer. They are excellent examples of the insidious nature of cancer and the result of a poor diet. Virtually everyone I spoke to who had had colorectal cancer detected in a routine physical said the same thing: "I never felt sick, nor did I feel a thing when the doctor said I had cancer. Now I live with a colostomy, which proves that you simply don't know."

Polyps are removed because 2.5 percent will become cancerous in five years, 8 percent in ten years, and 24 percent in twenty years. Once you have some polyps, it's a matter of time before one of them becomes cancerous. A study in the Burkitt tradition proved that fiber prevents polyps in the first place and helps return them to normal after they have developed.

At Cornell Medical Center, human volunteers who have and who develop polyps were chosen for a study. In addition to their regular diet, they ate a cereal twice daily that provides about 14 grams of hard wheat fiber. We'll discuss hard wheat fiber in chapter 7. A control group, matched by age, sex, and polyp tendency, ate a cereal that didn't have any fiber.

In six months, the people who got the hard wheat fiber had 30 percent fewer polyps than the members of the control group! A 30-percent reduction means that not only does the fiber prevent polyps, but some polyps disappear and the cells return to normal. This study has since been confirmed by other studies. With that news, why would you not have a high-fiber cereal every morning?

Think about that finding in human terms. About 150,000 people will be diagnosed with colorectal cancer this year. At least 50 percent and possibly as much as 90 percent of this cancer starts as a polyp. I'll say 50 percent to be conservative. That means at least 30 percent of 75,000 cases annually, or about 22,500 cases, could have been avoided by simply sitting down to a bowl of high-fiber cereal every day! Since only 37 percent of people who get bowel cancer survive five years, that's at least 14,175 lives that could have been saved in one year! Follow the high-fiber Longevity Diet in chapter 15. It pays big dividends.

BREAST CANCER: A BONUS

Everyone should know that the major risk factors for breast cancer are heredity, body fat, and dietary fat, although even alcohol has been implicated. These risks receive all the press, because they're easy to talk about. But how many times have you heard about constipation? That's right, simple constipation is a risk factor for cancer.

Breast cancer is thought to start, on average, because of byproducts of hormones the body makes itself. Elimination of these byproducts requires good circulation, regular exercise, plenty of water, and bowel regularity. Bowel regularity requires fiber and water, two nutrients that are an essential nutrition team.

Some statistics will make this point more obvious. One in ten American women gets breast cancer, and 23 percent of American women are constipated. That means that of one hundred women, twenty-three will be four times as likely to get breast cancer as the other seventy-seven, simply because their diet doesn't include enough fiber to make them have an easy movement every twenty-four to thirty-six hours that would eliminate hormonal byproducts.

When I talk to laypeople about fiber and regularity, they perk up and listen when I speak of fiber as nature's detoxifier. In the case of breast cancer, that's exactly how I envision fiber. It helps the body rid itself of toxins that increase the likelihood that some cell in the breast can become cancerous thanks to a material that's not eliminated quickly enough. The Longevity Diet has excellent prevention built into its fiber delivery.

FIBER DEFICIENCY IN THE 1990s

I wish I could tell you more encouraging stories about other cancers, like the ones on polyps or diverticulosis. Unfortunately, it's seldom that clear. People don't eat fiber; they eat food. So, most often, it's a dietary relationship with fruits, vegetables, and grains that counts. And there are other protector substances in those natural foods that also work, so it's never just one nutrient. However, there's no longer any doubt among scientists that fiber is important. Dennis Burkitt was correct. Many modern illnesses are fiber-deficiency diseases. I've summarized them in table 6.3.

TABLE 6.3

Fiber Deficiency Diseases

CANCER

Fiber Detoxifies Dietary Factors

- Colorectal cancer; stomach cancer
- Cancers in which regularity is important; these include stomach, pancreatic, breast, and prostate cancer

HEART DISEASE

A High-Fiber Diet Is a Low-Fat Diet

- Elevated blood fats including cholesterol and triglycerides
- High blood pressure

INTESTINAL DISORDERS

Fiber Helps to Tone the Intestine

- Gall bladder disease
- Irritable bowel disease
- Ileitis, colitis, and ulcerative colitis
- Appendicitis
- Inflammatory bowel diseases
- Diverticulosis
- Varicose veins and hemorrhoids

DIABETES MANAGEMENT

A High-Fiber Diet Is a Low-Sugar Diet

- Reduction and stabilization of blood sugar

In the next chapter you'll see how to get enough of the right kind of fiber to protect yourself from these diseases.

7

Protective
Fiber in Food

Most people don't understand fiber nor do they know how much they need or which foods they should eat to get enough. This chapter explains where to get fiber and even how to select fiber supplements. The following quiz identifies the salient points about dietary fiber in food.

Dietary Fiber Quiz

Answer yes or no to these questions:

- Do you eat a cereal daily that provides more than 4 grams of fiber?

- Do you eat hard to soft fiber in a ratio of 3 to 1?

- Do you use a fiber supplement?

- Do you know, within 10 percent, how much fiber your diet provides?

- Do you have an easy bowel movement every twenty-four to thirty-six hours?

132

A no to any of these questions indicates that you can improve your health options by learning about fiber from this chapter.

HOW MUCH FIBER DO YOU NEED?

Fiber need depends on the size of your digestive system. The more you weigh and the bigger you are, the more fiber you need.

Many years ago, health scientists settled on a 150-pound person as standard. Indeed, this seems a little chauvinistic, because it was probably a man, somewhat thin at that. However, it's convenient to think in those terms today and base recommendations proportionately. I recommend the following:

WEIGHT	MINIMUM FIBER	OPTIMUM FIBER
100 lbs.	20 grams	25 grams
125 lbs.	25 grams	30 grams
150 lbs.	30 grams	35 grams
175 lbs.	35 grams	40 grams
200 lbs.	40 grams	45 grams

Scientists don't all agree on how much fiber we should get in our diet; one panel of experts concluded that a 150-pound person needs about 30 grams daily, but another panel recommended 40 grams from evaluating the same scientific data. I set the optimum value as midway between these two recommendations and scaled the other amounts for other body weights from that.

As the twentieth century finishes its last decade, there aren't any serious health scientists who don't recognize the need for fiber. As you learned in the last chapter, it wasn't always this way, but now there's a meeting of the minds. Debate will always continue over what kinds of fiber are necessary, but these debates are in the realm of "crossing t's and dotting i's"; they aren't important to average people.

Now we realize that the seeds of some diseases, such as diverticulosis and cancer, are sown in youth. Consequently, parents reading this chapter can now take steps to increase the abundance of life for their children and grandchildren by simply applying the information they've read here.

A MAGIC FIBER RATIO

You know now that there are two broad types of fiber: soluble, or soft, fiber, and insoluble, or hard, fiber. The terms *soluble* and *insoluble* are being used more frequently on the labels of cereals and other processed foods, so I'll use them here. You should strive to get three times as much insoluble as soluble fiber and there's only one way to accomplish that—eat a variety of cereals, grains, vegetables, and fruit.

VARIETY: TEAMWORK

In nutrition, teamwork is essential. No nutrient, including fiber, works alone. In spite of all our knowledge, there's still more we don't know than know about fiber and health. Having a variety of fiber is the best way to achieve teamwork and overcome our ignorance.

Wheat bran improves regularity, but it doesn't lower cholesterol. Oat bran cereal and oatmeal lower cholesterol better than they improve regularity. Before you jump to eating only oat bran or oatmeal for cholesterol or wheat bran for regularity, remember from the last chapter that wheat bran also reduces polyps. There's one way out of the dilemma: learn to eat both types of cereals. You want low cholesterol, regularity, and no polyps. Practicing variety will help to accomplish this.

CHOLESTEROL LOWERING

In 1989, *The 8-Week Cholesterol Cure* by Robert E. Kowalski became a bestseller. It was based on the author's cholesterol-lowering experience with oatmeal and oat bran. Other scientists had discovered the same program in the 1950s, but the world wasn't ready to act on that knowledge. In 1989, the surgeon general said, "Lower your cholesterol to 200 milligrams per deciliter."

Oatmeal is a good source of soluble gums. These gums are excellent for removing bile acids, which, you learned in chapter 6, is the same as removing cholesterol from your blood. Can't stand oatmeal? There are other sources of gums and soluble fiber that will help lower cholesterol. Beans and other vegetables are excellent sources. At the end of this chapter, in table 8.4, you will find many sources of soluble fiber.

Fiber supplements are another approach to cholesterol lowering. Table 7.5 lists supplements made from gums, mucilage, and psyllium husks. By taking three to five grams of one of these fiber supplements at each meal, you can lower your cholesterol by as much as 20 percent in about two months.

BULK: REGULARITY

Table 7.1 illustrates how fiber from different sources influences our stools. Bulky, soft stools are regular stools. Study table 7.1 and you'll see that wheat bran, fruits, and vegetables increase stool volume most for each unit of fiber.

TABLE 7.1

Fiber Input Compared to Stool Output

Fiber Source or Type	Percentage of Stool Volume Increase Per Unit of Fiber	Cholesterol-Lowering Ability
Wheat Bran, raw or cooked	5.7	None
Fruits and vegetables: carrots, cabbage, peas, apple, beans, etc.	4.9	Fair
Oats: oat bran; rolled oats	3.9	Excellent
Gums and mucilages: psyllium, guar, sterculia	3.5	Excellent
Corn: corn bran, corn meal	3.4	Good
Cellulose, purified for paper	3.0	None
Soya fiber, bean hulls, pulp	2.8	Unknown
Pectin from fruit	1.3	Good

Now compare stool increase to the relative ability to lower cholesterol, the third column of table 7.1, and you can see why you need both types of fiber. Do you come to the same conclusion that I do? You need fiber from a wide variety of sources in order to get enough of both soluble and insoluble. I produced table 7.1 by analyzing results from many clinical studies. You will find more information in the reading list.

WHERE DO WE STAND?

Americans consume, on average, about 12 grams of fiber daily. Don't get the impression that we're irresponsible people; it's not our fault. The amount of fiber we take in has been declining for the last ten thousand years, since agriculture was developed.

In 1991, the problem is widespread. There's about 6.5 grams of fiber per 1,000 calories in the diet of average American women and 5.5 grams per 1,000 calories in the diet of most American men. A woman of 125 pounds needs 1,700 to 2,200 calories each day to stay trim and healthy. To get 30 grams of fiber from the average diet, she'd need 4,600 calories. She'd also weigh about 270 pounds at that level. Unless she's thinking of a career as a linebacker, she's got to make some dietary changes.

A man of 170 pounds needs from 2,200 to 2,500 calories daily. At 5.5 grams of fiber per 1,000 calories, he'd need about 5,400 calories; that's what a 170-pound, Olympic downhill-skier burns on the peak days of training. If most men ate 5,400 calories, they'd weigh about 360 pounds and be candidates for the couch potato Olympics.

These examples of how much fiber we get in average diets illustrate the modern dilemma. People used to be able to get that much fiber easily. Our ancestors worked harder physically and so needed to consume more calories. And their food had more fiber because it was less processed or refined. Since we no longer work as hard physically, we don't require as many calories. And as our caloric consumption declined, we shifted to a diet that was less bulky, as we exchanged fat and sugar for fiber. Now we can't possibly get sufficient fiber by simply eating more of the same food we've been eating. We will need to change our food and use fiber supplements.

WHAT HAPPENED?

In 1870, the roller mill let us make soft white flour, which, until then, had been very costly. The roller mill removed fiber from our breads, cakes, and other baked goods by crushing and removing the hulls or germs of grain, leaving only the white starchy parts of the grain.

Cold breakfast cereals were first introduced at the Battle Creek Clinic in the 1920s. These cereals were designed to increase dietary fiber in people with intestinal disorders, but somehow these cereals changed over time. The fiber came out of the cereal, and sugar was added. Sad to say, another major source of fiber disappeared.

Today, two people in five don't eat breakfast, unless you count toast or a roll with juice and coffee. Morning is the best time of day to easily get 6 or more grams of hard fiber from a high-fiber cereal; or you could get 3 to 4 grams from oatmeal, cracked wheat, or some other natural cereal.

But there's more. Over 30 percent of people have no fruit or, at most, they only have one serving during the day. Similarly, others don't eat vegetables more than once daily and there are many who don't even do that. Many young people identify salad as the garnish that comes with a burger. There's no way these people will ever get enough fiber if they don't change their eating habits or use fiber supplements.

A major fiber decline has come from fast food. Most fast-food outlets provide food that is rich in calories, often supplying as much as 50 percent of a person's daily calories in one meal (hamburger, fries, and a shake) with only a couple grams of fiber at best. Unless the other 50 percent of daily calories are carefully thought out, individuals who eat this way will never come close to getting even half the fiber they need.

FIBER REQUIRES SOME CHANGES

Getting enough fiber simply requires some changes in food selection. These changes will become habit, you'll feel better, and then you'll wonder how you ever ate any other way. Increase the fiber you get from food, and you'll automatically cut fat out of your diet. An easy approach is to simply follow the Longevity Diet in chapter 15.

FIBER IN: FAT OUT

Getting fat out is simple. It calls for remembering a few rules. I can't tell you what to eat every day, but I can tell you where the fat resides. Remember, most fat is hidden. Write these rules on a card and carry it with you:

- Fast food is fat food!
- Red meat is fat meat!
- Fried food is fat food!
- Baked goods and candy are fat food!
- Cheese and sauces make good food fat!
- Booze is fat food!
- Bulky, natural food is good food!

You don't have to cut out all the fat foods, but you've got to eat them sparingly. There's a motto I like to use when counseling people about eating: Don't waste calories! Eliminate foods that don't contribute to your health unless you've been saving calories for the occasion.

Think before you eat. Why not save some calories for a glass of wine with dinner or a reasonable dessert? The reward is worth it: You'll live longer and better, the roses will smell sweeter, and think of how regular you'll become.

GETTING THE RIGHT FIBER

I've broken the sources of fiber into foods you can adapt to easily. We'll start with cereals, then look at vegetables and fruits. You'll see that there's fiber all around us, and the objective of 30 grams a day is easily within your grasp.

Cereals

Table 7.2 identifies cereals that deliver enough fiber. Any cereal that delivers 4 or more grams of fiber per serving is acceptable. If you have cereal in your closet with less than 4 grams per serving, there's only one thing to do: Feed it to the birds and don't buy it again! You might be surprised, because the birds often won't eat these cereals.

A few cereals deliver as much as 14 grams of fiber. They're excellent, but you've got to work up to them or mix them with other cereals that deliver about 4 grams per serving to start. Going from very little fiber at a meal, or 12 grams in a whole day, to 14 grams in one meal is too much for most people. Work up to that level in a few meals.

TABLE 7.2

High Fiber Cereals

Product Name	Manufacturer	Fiber Content in grams		Total
		Soluble	Insoluble	
VERY HIGH FIBER				
HEARTWISE (psyllium added)	KELLOGGS	4	3	7
FIBER ONE	GENERAL MILLS	Not declared		13
100% BRAN WITH OAT BRAN	NABISCO	Not declared		8
100% BRAN	NABISCO	2	8	10
100% NATURAL OAT BRAN	ESCONDIDO MILLS	4	8	12
HIGH FIBER CEREALS				
FRUITFUL BRAN	KELLOGGS	Not declared		
MUSLIX	KELLOGGS	Not declared		4
CRACKLIN OAT BRAN	KELLOGGS	Not declared		4
BRAN FLAKES	KELLOGGS	Not declared		5

HIGH FIBER CEREALS

40% BRAN FLAKES	SAFEWAY (Store brand)	Not declared	4
RAISIN BRAN	KELLOGGS	Not declared	5
RAISIN BRAN	SAFEWAY (Store brand)	Not declared	4
FRUIT 'N FIBRE	POST	Not declared	5
TOTAL RAISIN BRAN	GENERAL MILLS	Not declared	5
SHREDDED WHEAT 'N BRAN	NABISCO	1	3	4
SHREDDED WHEAT WITH OAT BRAN	NABISCO	1	3	4
MAYPO- OATMEAL WITH ADDED BRAN (cooked cereal)	AMERICAN HOME FOODS	Not declared	4
OAT BRAN	QUAKER	Not declared	4
INSTANT OAT BRAN	NABISCO	2	3	5
CRUNCHY BRAN	QUAKER	Not declared	5
WHEATENA (cooked cereal)	AMERICAN HOME FOODS	Not declared	4

You may not find all the products listed in table 7.2 in your supermarket because brands and products change from month to month, but the cereals in table 7.2 are fairly consistent and are likely to stay. Just learn to read labels, and don't eat a cereal unless it delivers at least 4 grams of fiber per serving. A large supermarket has approximately twenty-five thousand, constantly changing choices to select from, so it's better to follow these three rules than to expect the foods to remain unchanged.

- Don't eat a cereal with less than 4 grams of fiber per serving.

- The cereal should have at least 2 grams of hard or insoluble fiber.

- Strive for over 7 grams of fiber per serving.

Fruits

Myriad fresh fruit exist in this great country. In other chapters we'll talk about the other protector substances fruit provides. A good point to remember is that fiber content varies with variety, season, and climate, so you always get an estimate. It's another reason why variety is so important.

TABLE 7.3

Fruit Sources of Fiber

| Food | Serving Size | Fiber Content Per Serving, in Grams | | |
		Soluble	Insoluble	Total
Apple	1 medium	0.8	2.0	2.8
Apricot	2 small	0.7	0.8	1.5
Banana	1 medium	0.6	1.4	2.0
Blackberries	1 cup	1.4	7.6	9.0
Cherries	10	0.3	0.9	1.2
Grapefruit	½ medium	0.6	1.1	1.7
Grapes	12	0.1	0.4	0.5
Orange	1 medium	0.5	1.3	1.8
Peach	1 medium	0.6	1.0	1.6
Pear	1 medium	1.0	4.0	5.0
Pineapple	1 cup	0.6	1.8	2.4
Plum	3 small	0.7	1.1	1.8
Raspberries	1 cup	0.5	8.3	8.8
Strawberries	1 cup	0.9	1.7	2.6

These data are taken from various sources. The values here may differ from those seen elsewhere because values vary according to variety, season, location, and method of measurement.

For more comprehensive information, consult the reading list.

Think of fruit as an excellent source of snack and dessert and as an ingredient for cooking. I'm normally opposed to processed food, except when it comes to fiber from fruits and vegetables. Frozen and canned fruits and vegetables contain as much fiber as their raw counterparts. The only loss is when the skin is removed for canning. People with inflammatory bowel diseases actually do better on canned foods, as I explained in *Eating Right for a Bad Gut.*

Vegetables

Types of vegetables are even more numerous than fruit. Table 7.4 lists typical vegetables in the same way table 7.3 listed fruit. If a vegetable isn't listed, you can estimate its fiber content from another similar vegetable. As you inspect table 7.4, think back to tables 7.2 and 7.3 to visualize how you'd get 30 grams of fiber daily.

TABLE 7.4

Vegetable Sources of Fiber

| Food | Serving Size | Fiber Content Per Serving, in Grams | | |
		Soluble	Insoluble	Total
Asparagus	¾ cup	0.8	2.3	3.1
Beans:				
Green	½ cup	0.5	1.6	2.1
Kidney	½ cup	2.5	3.3	5.8
Lima	½ cup	1.2	3.2	4.4
Pinto	½ cup	2.0	3.3	5.3
White	½ cup	1.4	3.6	5.0
Broccoli	½ cup	0.9	1.1	2.0
Brussels sprouts	½ cup	1.6	2.3	3.9
Cabbage	½ cup	0.9	1.1	2.0
Carrots	½ cup	1.1	1.2	2.3
Cauliflower	½ cup	0.5	1.1	1.6
Celery	½ cup	0.4	0.9	1.3
Corn	½ cup	1.7	2.2	3.9
Eggplant	½ cup	0.8	1.2	2.0
Kale	½ cup	1.4	1.4	2.8
Lettuce	½ cup	0.1	0.2	0.3
Onions	½ cup	0.8	1.8	2.6
Peas	½ cup	1.1	3.0	4.1
Potatoes, baked:				
Sweet	½ cup	0.7	1.0	1.7
White	½ cup	0.9	0.9	1.8
Radishes	5 medium	0.1	0.5	0.6

Squash:

Acorn	½ cup	0.5	3.8	4.3
Zucchini	½ cup	1.3	1.4	2.7
Tomato	1 medium	0.2	0.6	0.8
Turnip	½ cup	0.8	0.9	1.7
Almonds	1 tablespoon	0.1	1.0	1.1

These data are estimated from various sources.

There is still much debate about methods of measuring dietary fiber and about the difference between soluble and insoluble fibers. Don't be concerned if these numbers differ from others you have seen, because the values are not precise.

Grains and Breads

Breads and muffins made from whole grain are acceptable sources of fiber. If a bread doesn't provide 1 gram of fiber per slice or two grams in one muffin, don't eat it! Don't waste calories on food without fiber. Save the calories for a little treat like a glass of decent wine, or a special dessert or snack. And if the label doesn't declare the fiber content, don't purchase the product!

Fiber Supplements

Thanks to the marvels of engineering, you can purchase excellent fiber supplements. Perhaps the most familiar is Metamucil. Metamucil is typical of a soluble fiber supplement. It's made from psyllium husks, and one teaspoon supplies 3.4 grams of fiber. Metamucil is mucilage and is excellent at lowering cholesterol. Many stores stock their own generic copy of Metamucil labeled as vegetable laxative. These products are similarly made from psyllium husks and are similar to Metamucil.

The only rule is that the supplement should provide over three grams of fiber in a convenient serving. Be sure you purchase a fiber supplement and not a powdered laxative.

TABLE 7.5

Fiber Supplements

Product	Company	Type of Fiber
Metamucil	Procter & Gamble	Soluble fiber from psyllium husk
Fiberall	Rydell Labs Inc.	Soluble fiber from psyllium husk
Daily Fiber Blend	Shaklee Corporation	Blend of soluble and insoluble fiber
Fiber Plan	Shaklee Corporation	Special blend of soluble fiber to lower cholesterol
Vegetable Laxative	Generic Store Brands	Soluble fiber from psyllium husk

A DAY IN THE LIFE OF FIBER

I've provided two days' worth of menus to show you how you can eat 35 grams of fiber without using fiber supplements. You can use these examples or create your own. In the tabulations, I've included calories; then I've shown you how you can add in the entrees with their caloric delivery.

I've selected all the foods from the tables in this chapter. Notice that I added extra calories for spreads and condiments. For the sake of this book, I didn't mention the garlic and onions that go with fish and meat. I usually have some beans, but the vegetable variety is more than adequate.

These menus prove it can be done with enough calories left over for alternatives, including beverages. There's no excuse for falling into the typical American habit of only 12 grams of fiber daily. Either diet plan, if followed regularly, will keep weight and cholesterol down and allows ample room for snacks.

TABLE 7.6

Menu for a Day of Fiber

Food	FIBER, IN GRAMS		Total	Calories
	Soluble	Insoluble		
BREAKFAST				
Bran Flakes, 1 ounce	1.0	4.0	5.0	121
(with ½ cup 2% milk)				93
½ grapefruit	0.6	1.1	1.7	39
SNACK				
Banana	0.6	1.4	2.0	105
LUNCH				
2 slices wheat bread	0.6	2.2	2.8	122
Corn, ½ cup	1.7	2.2	3.9	89
Broccoli, ½ cup	1.6	2.3	3.9	23
Peach (dessert), 1 medium	0.6	1.0	1.6	37
SNACK				
Apple, 1 medium	0.8	2.0	2.8	81
DINNER				
Brussels sprouts, ½ cup	1.6	2.3	3.9	30
Small salad	1.6	2.2	3.8	50
Potato, medium baked	0.7	1.0	1.7	200
Melon (dessert), ¼	0.4	0.6	1.0	130
SNACK				
Pear, 1 medium	0.5	2.0	2.5	98
Total	12.3	24.3	35.6	1218

Other foods eaten during the day:

	Calories
Yogurt	228
Turkey slices, 2 ounces (lunch)	100
Fish, 2 ounces (dinner)	150
Spreads and condiments	100
Total calories	578
Total daily calories	1796

This day is designed to provide enough fiber, with a little flexibility. There's room for most people to have desserts or accompaniments, such as wine.

TABLE 7.7

Menu for a Day of High Fiber and Low Calories

Food	FIBER, IN GRAMS Soluble	Insoluble	Total	Calories
BREAKFAST				
Fiber One, 1 ounce	1.0	12.0	13.0	60
(with ½ cup skim milk)				40
½ Grapefruit	0.6	1.1	1.7	39
SNACK				
Apple, 1 medium	0.8	2.0	2.8	81
LUNCH				
Corn, ½ cup	1.7	2.2	3.9	89
Broccoli, ½ cup	1.6	2.3	3.9	23
Banana, 1 medium	0.6	1.4	2.0	105

DINNER

Eggplant, ½ cup	0.8	1.2	2.0	45
Small salad	1.6	2.2	3.8	50
Melon (dessert), ¼	0.4	0.6	1.0	130
Total	9.1	26.2	35.3	662

Other foods eaten during the day:

	Calories
Yogurt	228
Fish (lunch)	150
Steak (dinner)	250
Spreads, dressings, and condiments	100
Total calories	728
Total daily calories	1390

This day is designed for a person watching calories. At 1,390 total calories, flexibility remains for wine, dessert, or even a snack, such as a bagel, and it provides 35 grams of fiber.

SUMMARY

While the average diet provides 6 grams of fiber per 1,000 calories, you can get 35 grams in 2,000 calories or over 17.5 grams of fiber per 1,000 calories. That's the level necessary to obtain the protective effects of dietary fiber. A few rules apply:

- Eat high-fiber cereal daily (cereals with over 10 grams of fiber are conveniently available).

- Eat fruit at every meal.

- Eat vegetables at every meal.

- Eat vegetables or fruit for snacks.

- Use fiber supplements to make up shortfalls.

- Don't waste calories.

8

Balancing Essential Oils

The common expression "Fish is brain food" comes to us from ancient China and the early Christian era of the Western world. This saying, over two thousand years old, reemerged in the early nineteenth century when German scientists discovered that phosphorus was essential for energy. These scientists said, "No phosphorus, no thought," because thinking requires energy.

About 1850, American naturalist Alexander Agassiz observed that fish is rich in phosphorus and said once again, "Fish is brain food." His comment encouraged people to eat fish, so it was an important announcement. Both the German scientists and Agassiz were correct in their conclusions, but for the wrong reason. Fish is brain food because of an essential oil, not because of phosphorus.

Fish supplies a critical oil, docosahexaenoic acid (DHA), that is essential for brain and eye tissue development in infants and children and is essential for maintaining these tissues throughout life. Breast milk contains a significant amount of DHA, which is passed to the nursing infant. This nutrient alone is a good reason for women to breastfeed their children. Since DHA is such an important nutrient in brain and eye development, it truly is brain food, and fish is the most practical source. So, once again, folk wisdom is correct.

148

Essential Oils Quiz

Answer yes or no to the following questions:

- Have you or any blood relative had an inflammatory disease such as arthritis, psoriasis, Crohn's disease, or asthma?

- Do you or any blood relative get frequent migraine headaches?

- Have you or a blood relative had a stroke? High blood pressure?

- Have you or any blood relative had cancer (not including lung cancer), especially breast cancer?

- Have you or any blood relative developed diabetes where insulin is required?

Learn more about how essential oils help prevent these diseases.

DISCOVERING THE OIL PROTECTORS

In the early 1930s, a biochemist named Von Euler discovered a substance in human semen that makes a woman's vagina contract in wavelike spasms. He and his collaborators uncovered the structure of this substance, which comes from the prostate gland, and named it prostaglandin. This was just the beginning. Another biochemist, Dr. John Vane, dedicated forty years to prostaglandin research and identified three prostaglandins. In 1982, Dr. Vane shared the Nobel Prize in Physiology and Medicine for this and subsequent discoveries about the prostaglandins. Now we know that there are more than three prostaglandins and several large subgroups of each one that regulate many body functions.

Prostaglandins are produced within each active cell of our body when circumstances call for them, circumstances such as mucous secretion, inflammation, tonicity of blood vessels, flexibility of blood cells, immune-system function, and the inflammation or tightening of blood vessels to control blood pressure. This means that when our body is functioning correctly, we can make the right prostaglandins when they are needed to regulate a function or to help the body defend itself.

It follows that the substances from which prostaglandins are made must be available in the correct amounts and in the right balance. Since prostaglandins are made from the essential oils, that is where we must focus our attention. We obtain the essential oils from our diet to gain the protection of the prostaglandins.

We'll start by taking a short lesson in fats.

FATS

Fat is nature's most concentrated source of energy and should be about 20 percent of total calories; between 20 and 30 percent of our calories as fat is optimum. The Longevity Diet in chapter 15 achieves this amount very nicely. Dietary fat contains three broad groups according to their structure. We call these three groups saturated fats, monounsaturated fats, and polyunsaturated fats.

You've already encountered these three groups in your kitchen and supermarket. It's helpful to visualize them.

• Saturated fat is hard at room temperature. Two good examples are butter and the white fat around a steak's red meat. Both are hard at room temperature even though butter will melt at about 100 degrees.

• Monounsaturated fat is usually an amber liquid at room temperature, gets cloudy in the refrigerator, and is hard in the freezer. Olive oil is an excellent readily available example. Put a small glass of olive oil in the refrigerator and one in the freezer, and you'll see what I mean. They're both still usable after their cold experience.

• Polyunsaturated fat is a clear light liquid at room temperature; it stays clear in the refrigerator and won't harden in most home freezers. Corn oil and safflower oil are good examples.

Natural oils and fats are really a mixture of all three types of fat in which one type predominates. So beef fat is mostly saturated fat, but contains some mono- and polyunsaturated fats. Similarly, olive oil is mostly monounsaturated fat with polyunsaturated fat and a little saturated fat. Corn oil is mostly polyunsaturated fat with some monounsaturated fat and very little saturated fat.

Our focus now, however, is on polyunsaturated fats because the essential oils, the protectors, are all polyunsaturated fats and fall into two large groups.

ESSENTIAL OILS

Polyunsaturated fatty acids occur in one of two basic chemical structures that chemists identify as omega-3 and omega-6. This international method of naming them is based on their structure and helps chemists distinguish one group of polyunsaturated oils from the other. You just need to recognize that there are three oils in each group. Since the oils in each group are related to each other, I think of them as families. It's important to know why you need them and how you can get them.

I know that family trees can be complex, but each family tree of essential oils is very simple. Each essential oil family has three members that differ from one another only by small increments in size, even though it's at a level we can't see with the best electron microscope. Each member of every family is important, because alone they either produce a critical prostaglandin or are essential to health. For example, in the omega-3 family, one oil, EPA, produces a critical prostaglandin, while the next oil in the family, DHA, is crucial to brain and eye development ("fish is brain food").

Fish require omega-3 oils for body function at cold temperatures, which is one reason we find the omega-3 oils in fish. Fish oils, mostly omega-3s, don't solidify until minus 103 degrees Fahrenheit, and the colder the water, the more oils the fish has. Fish are cold-blooded, which means they take on the temperature of the water they live in. In contrast, corn oil, mostly omega-6s, solidifies at minus 4 degrees. Some cold-water fish swim in salt water that would immobilize land mammals even if they could survive it. Marine mammals that also inhabit the cold waters, such as whales and sea lions, have oils similar to those of fish and not to those of land animals. Since polar bears live mostly on fish and sea mammals, their flesh is similarly rich in these oils.

Sources of the omega-3 oils are generally very different from those for omega-6 oils, although, as is often true for biological materials, some of both groups of oils are always found together. The large difference between their solidifying temperatures helps us identify the various sources of these oils.

All green plants, such as grasses and leaves, contain some omega-3 oils. Algae in the cold ocean or fresh water are the most abundant sources by weight. Since fish eat algae and need oils that become solid only at an extremely low temperature, fish concentrate omega-3 oils. In fact, the colder the water, the more omega-3 oils the fish contain. We also find omega-3 oils in some seeds from colder growing regions, such as flaxseed and rapeseed, and nuts that grow on trees, such as walnuts and almonds. One green plant, purslane, is rich in omega-3 oils.

Grains such as corn and oil-bearing beans such as soy are rich in omega-6 oils. Since we fatten beef on corn and raise cows on grain, we get omega-6 oils in beef and animal products, such as milk. Further, since corn and soy oils are so widely used in food processing, you find omega-6 in most processed foods from bread to salad oils.

In contrast to present-day eating habits, when people regularly ate game, such as rabbits and venison, they did get a good balance of both groups of oils. This is because the grasses, nuts, and berries these foraging animals eat contain a correct balance of the two groups of oils. Also, since their flesh is much lower in fat, diets didn't have as much fat and the fat was more correctly balanced in omega-3 and omega-6 oils.

TWO FAMILIES OF ESSENTIAL OILS

The simplest omega-3 oil is called alpha linolenic acid (ALA). The simplest omega-6 oil is called linoleic acid; it has no abbreviation. At one time, linoleic acid was proposed for vitamin status but rejected for technical reasons, so you can see how important it is. Our essential oil requirement can be satisfied by getting these two oils, ALA and linoleic acid, from our diet.

Once you've gotten either ALA and linoleic acids in your diet, your body can build the rest of each group of oils, illustrated in table 8.1. I've also listed the common dietary sources for each oil.

TABLE 8.1

Common Dietary Sources of Omega-3 and Omega-6 Oils

Omega-3 Family	Omega-6 Family
Alpha Linolenic Acid (ALA) Seed oils: flaxseed, soy, rapeseed, Canola oil, green plants, nuts (metabolism) ↓ in body	*Linoleic Acid* Corn oil, soybean oil, and other vegetable oils ↓ (metabolism) in body
Eicosapentaenoic Acid (EPA) Cold-water fish, marine mammals ↓ (metabolism) in body	*Gamma Linolenic Acid (GLA)* Seed oils: oil of evening primrose, black-currant seed oil ↓ (metabolism) in body
Docasahexaenoic Acid (DHA) Fish, marine mammals	*Arachidonic Acid (AA)* Meat, animal fat, animal products (e.g., milk, butter)

Table 8.1 illustrates that ALA is generally obtained from seed oils that are not widely eaten. ALA is also found in green plants, including the algae of the oceans and lakes, and purslane, which grows on land. Nut sources include almonds and walnuts, but not the peanut, which is really a legume. The next two members of the group, eicosapentaenoic acid (EPA) and docosahexaenoic acid (DHA), are readily obtained from fish and marine mammals.

Fish eat green algae and make EPA and DHA, which are required for their tissues. These oils aren't solid at minus 103 degrees, so they are essential to coldwater fish. Without question, fish and marine mammals, such as sea lions and whales, are the best sources of these oils.

Look at table 8.1 again and you'll see that there are many common sources of linoleic acid and arachidonic acid (AA). For example, we use corn oil or other vegetable oils to cook, or bake, in processing foods, in salad dressings, and in most aspects of food preparation. Further, we get lots of AA from meat, dairy products, and any other animal-based food.

However, the intermediate oil, gamma linolenic acid (GLA), is generally not obtained in foods. Who eats primrose seeds or black currants? It's safe to conclude that our diet contains very little, if any, GLA, even though our body makes some. In the future, GLA could be more important than it now appears. The next short chapter will cover this.

IS BALANCING THE OILS IMPORTANT?

Jorn Dyerberg, a Danish epidemiologist, knew from general information that Greenlanders ate a high-fat diet exceptionally rich in the omega-3 oils, and the Danes, their genetic ancestors, ate a similarly high-fat diet very rich in omega-6 oils. The groups had about the same amount of fat in their diet as ours in the United States, which is similar to the Danes.

Dyerberg also knew that the Greenlanders didn't seem to have the same diseases that we and the Danes share, such as heart disease, arthritis, and high blood pressure. Dyerberg felt these two populations were an excellent starting place to settle, once and for all, the importance of the balance of the omega-3 and omega-6 oils in health.

Genetics was another reason, besides diet, that the Dane-Greenlander comparison was especially good. If Dyerberg found some major differences, he didn't want people to say: "How do you know it's not just heredity?" He could say, with unusual accuracy, that both groups came from the same genetic stock.

The study he undertook has already served as a monument of what a careful epidemiologist can discover. He and his group lived among Greenlanders, cooked their food as they do, mixed it, and analyzed it. They had to work under uncomfortable conditions compared to their nice, warm, modern, well-equipped labs in Denmark. We all owe a salute to these men of science.

OUR DIETARY FAT

Dyerberg didn't stop at a superficial comparison by asking people to keep a diary of what they ate. He actually took their food and analyzed it. This step was critical, because he could exactly define their omega-3 and omega-6 oil intake very precisely. It also established a baseline for the next step, which was analyzing their blood.

In table 8.2 I've compared the dietary fat of Danes to that of their Greenlander counterparts. This data collected by Jorn Dyerberg shows that the Greenlander diet favors the omega-3 oils and the Danish diet favors the omega-6 oils.

TABLE 8.2

Dietary Fat Composition

Dietary Fat	Danes	Greenlanders
Percentage of calories from fat	42	39
Percentage of saturated fat	53	23
Percentage of monounsaturated fat	34	58
Percentage of polyunsaturated fat	13	19
Total cholesterol, in milligrams	420	700
Ratio of polyunsaturated to saturated fat	0.2	0.8
Daily Intake:		
Omega-3, in grams	3	14
Omega-6, in grams	10	5
Ratio of omega-6 to omega-3	3.3	0.4

Table 8.2 makes several points very clear, and they're important to consider:

- Both diets are extremely high in fat. They exceed all Heart Association recommendations, which suggest keeping fat to less than 30 percent of calories. The Longevity Diet easily goes below the 30 percent level.

- Greenlanders and Danes exceed the recommended daily limit of 300 milligrams of cholesterol by a stretch. The Greenlanders eat even more cholesterol than the Danes.

- The ratio of polyunsaturated fat to saturated fat shows that the Greenlander diet is slightly richer in polyunsaturated fat than the Danes' diet.

- The ratio of the omega-6 to omega-3 oils proves that the Greenlanders' diet is far richer in omega-3 than omega-6 oils.

Dyerberg expected, in fact, hoped to find this result, because the Greenlanders eat fish and marine mammals.

As an aside, our American diet, as well as the Canadian and English diets, are the same as the Danes' diet. Most European countries have a similar diet; the exceptions being parts of Italy and Greece, the Faeroe Islands, and a few other areas.

If you didn't know any more about these two groups of people, you'd expect both of them to have a high rate of heart disease. You might even predict that the Greenlanders would be worse off than the Danes because of their cholesterol intake. Dyerberg carefully took a look at their blood fats. After all, diets can be misinterpreted and people can lie, but blood analysis gives a true picture of what people have been eating. You really are what you eat.

Dyerberg did very careful blood fat analyses on everyone in the study. He verified that what they said they ate, and what he saw them eat, was confirmed by body composition. In short, they were what they ate. Table 8.3 confirms very vividly that both groups ate as they said.

TABLE 8.3

Blood Fat Composition of Danes and Greenlanders

| Oil | Danes | | Greenlanders | |
	Percentage	Ratio*	Percentage	Ratio*
		BLOOD		
Omega-6**	30.7		8.0	
		7.4		0.7
Omega-3***	4.0		11.0	
		PLATELETS		
Omega-6**	30.3		12.4	
		15.0		0.9
Omega-3***	2.0		13.8	

*Ratio is defined as the omega-6 total divided by the omega-3 total.
**Omega-6 figure is the sum of linoleic acid and arachidonic acid (AA).
***Omega-3 figure is the sum of EPA and DHA.

Blood composition confirmed very clearly what the diets had predicted. The Greenlanders' blood was much richer in the omega-3 oils than the omega-6 oils; and their presence in the blood platelets, which change their composition very slowly, confirmed their eating habits were a long-standing dietary trend, not something the Greenlanders had eaten a day or so before. With this information as a foundation, Dyerberg could analyze the differences in health between Greenlanders and Danes to see if the difference in their diets produced obvious effects on their health.

DIET-RELATED HEALTH DIFFERENCES

I've summarized the Dyerberg health observations in table 8.4.

TABLE 8.4

Relative Health Differences Between Danes and Greenlanders

Disease	Incidence Among Danes	Incidence Among Greenlanders
Heart attack	XXXXX	X
Stroke	XX	XXXX
Psoriasis	XXXXX	X
Diabetes	XXXXX	None
Asthma	XXXXX	None
Thyroid toxicosis	XXXXX	X
Multiple sclerosis	XXXXX	None
Epilepsy	X	XX
Rheumatoid arthritis	XXXXX	X
Ulcers	XXXXX	XX
Cancer	XXXXX	XXX
Breast cancer	XXXXX	None
Inflammatory bowel disease	XXXX	None

X is a measurable level.
XX is definite and consistent signs of the disease.
XXX is average occurrence of the disease.
XXXX is high incidence of the disease.
XXXXX is very high incidence of the disease.

There are several striking features that stand out. Let me summarize them for you:

- *Heart attack:* Greenlanders have far fewer than their Danish counterparts. By comparison to ours or Danish societies, heart attacks are not an issue in their society.

- *Stroke:* Greenlanders die of stroke more than any other cause. Their rate is twice the Danish rate. It's not a major cause of death in Denmark, so the rate among Greenlanders is comparatively high.

- *Diabetes:* The incidence among the Greenlanders is too low to accurately measure. It affects about 6 percent of the Danish people, which is a rate similar to that in other countries; not so with the Greenlanders. For example, in the United States, diabetes affects over 6 percent of the population and the number is growing.

- *Arthritis:* The Greenlanders' rate is also less than 4 percent of the Danes' rate. It's even lower for inflammatory, auto-immune, and bowel diseases, such as colitis and Crohn's disease. In fact, this single observation has already led to some changes in treating those diseases. Researchers would expect these illnesses to be the same or higher than in Denmark because of the severe climate.

- *Psoriasis:* Psoriasis is one of many inflammatory diseases you'd expect among the Greenlanders, but it doesn't exist.

- *Epilepsy:* The Greenlanders' rate is about twice the Danes' rate. We'll come back to this, because it gives insight into excesses.

- *Multiple sclerosis (MS):* MS doesn't exist among the Greenlanders. This is another autoimmune disease that you could expect to see in their climate because the stress of very cold weather frequently brings it on.

- *Asthma:* Another inflammatory disease that occurs at about 4 percent of the rate in Denmark and other developed countries. Due to the severe climate, you'd expect a high rate among the Greenlanders.

- *Primary hypothyroidism (also called thyroidtoxicosis or a low-*

thyroid activity): This is usually considered an autoimmune disease in which thyroid-hormone production is inadequate. The Greenlanders' rate is about 4 percent of the rate for Danes or North Americans.

- *Ulcer:* Greenlanders have ulcers at about 34 percent of the rate that affects the Danes. This is a 66-percent reduction, if viewed from the Danish point of view. In hindsight, this difference could have been predicted.

- *Cancer (omitting breast cancer):* Although it's not completely correct to lump all cancer together, we'll do it here to make some points later. The Greenlander cancer rate is about 84 percent of the Danish rate. Seen another way, it's a 16-percent reduction. This has since been confirmed by direct animal experimentation.

- *Breast cancer:* It doesn't exist among the Greenlanders!

- *Inflammatory bowel disease:* It doesn't exist among the Greenlanders!

Dyerberg's research was very thorough. He completely eliminated the variable of heredity and raised important issues. In spite of that, the first question other scientists raised was: Does it apply anywhere but in Greenland?

CONFIRMATION OF THE GREENLANDER EXPERIENCE

Confirmation of Dyerberg's research has come from studies done on genetically homogeneous people, such as the Japanese, and genetically nonhomogeneous people, such as the Dutch, Americans, and Italians. These studies have included locations such as Japan, Holland, the Faeroe Islands, Alaska, Italy, the United States, and Canada. Some studies have included dietary changes, either by having people who don't normally do so eat fish or by having them take fish-oil supplements. All these studies have confirmed Dyerberg's original findings. Some findings deserve more mention because they have broader implications.

BREAST CANCER: A FUTURE CHALLENGE

A finding that persists unchallenged in Dyerberg's and other scientists' research is the remarkable difference in the rates of breast cancer. Dyerberg's original research (table 8.4) showed that the Greenlanders have no breast cancer. Research on the other societies that eat a great deal of fish has verified his findings by turning up either no breast cancer or a very low rate compared to the rate in no-fish eaters. The question is: "How can this be?" No one really knows for sure, but some scientists have a good idea of where to look.

Cancer cells are invaders that grow from within when something goes awry. Just as the body produces white blood cells to attack foreign invaders, like bacteria and viruses, the body produces killer cells to attack cancer cells. Some scientists call them "Pac-Man" cells in an analogy to the video game in which the good guys gobble up the bad guys and the game is for the good guys to win. That's the way the killer cells are supposed to work against cancer cells.

One hypothesis teaches that when breast cancer is in its very early stages, the Pac-Man cells don't attack the early cancer cells as they should; it has something to do with their inability to recognize cancer cells as the enemy. They make a mistake of omission.

Is the Pac-Man mistake similar to the mistake made in autoimmune diseases? In autoimmune diseases, Pac-Man cells selectively attack the body's own tissues. No one knows for sure why they do this. As scientists delve deeper into the complex biochemistry of immunity, prostaglandins, autoimmune diseases, and reasons why cancer cells can grow unattacked, we will find an answer. We can't leave Dyerberg's findings about cancer, especially breast cancer, until the differences that result from diet alone, which he and other researchers have identified, are explained.

Dyerberg's findings are compelling evidence that the omega-3 oils are a cancer preventive. However, his findings are much more widely accepted now because direct animal experimentation can be added in support of them. Dr. William T. Cave, Jr., of the University of Rochester has critically examined all the supportive animal studies and concluded that the omega-3 oils are definitely a cancer preventive. But Cave goes a step further and concludes there is evidence that these oils have a curative effect after a tumor has been established. This confirms the far-reaching implications of Dyerberg's research for the role of diet on health. See the reading list if you care to pursue this further.

A NAGGING DIFFERENCE: STROKE AND EPILEPSY

Several reasons are given for the higher rate of stroke among Greenlanders. Even though smoking wasn't accounted for in the study, it does increase the risk of heart disease and stroke, but the rate of heart disease was down while that for strokes was up. The spectacular reduction in heart disease in the Greenlanders has no influence on their tendency to have strokes. But the high fish-oil diet increases clotting time; that is, their blood doesn't clot as quickly.

One hypothesis that now has research support states that when an internal blood clot does form in Greenlanders, it is larger, more devastating, and more likely to find its way into the capillaries of the brain than blood clots formed by blood that clots more quickly. Other studies have proven the Greenlanders' experience with stroke is not typical of people who balance the omega-3 and omega-6 oils equally and not three to one as they do. Stroke seems to be high only among people eating large quantities of marine mammals, such as sea lions, whales, and walruses. In this regard, the Greenlanders' diet is probably too high in the omega-3 oils. Other studies support this hypothesis.

Epilepsy is not sufficiently widespread among either Danes or Greenlanders for Dyerberg's findings to be conclusive. However, the increased rate strongly suggests that the Greenlanders' diet could be excessive in omega-3 oils. This observation taken with the stroke experience implies that the fat balance has been tipped too far in the omega-3 direction by the Greenlanders. The increased incidence of epilepsy is the only other finding in Dyerberg's data that was not supported in other studies.

Both Dyerberg's study and experiments with taurine suggest that epilepsy can be markedly influenced by diet. So Dyerberg's study helps to open another avenue of research into this terrible disease. It underscores the fact that balancing the essential oils is an important dietary criterion.

PROSTAGLANDINS AS REGULATORS OF HEALTH

Dyerberg's discoveries brought into focus the body of knowledge that had its beginnings in 1934, when Von Euler discovered prostaglandin. Since Von Euler's discovery, three prostaglandins—PGE_1, PGE_2, and PGE_3—continue to be an area of intense research. Prostaglandins are made by all the cells of our body except by red blood cells. Understanding the prostaglandins has helped us see how subtleties of our health are regulated. They are described by some scientists as hormonelike and by others as cellular messengers; they're both.

Prostaglandins regulate body functions by causing each cell in any tissue to act in unison. They do this directly in some cases and by producing other, more active materials called leukotrienes, in other cases. The actual mechanisms by which the prostaglandins and leukotrienes exert their influence is at the cutting edge of modern biochemical research. As this research unfolds, it is opening more vistas for unlocking the cause of disease.

Prostaglandins are made from the oils EDA, GLA, and AA, which we've been discussing. Each one is made by the body from one of three oils as follows:

Linoleic Acid

$\downarrow$

Omega-6 oils   Gamma Linolenic Acid (GLA) $\rightarrow PGE_1$

$\downarrow$

Arachidonic Acid (AA) $\rightarrow PGE_2$

_____

Alpha Linolenic Acid (ALA)

$\downarrow$

Omega-3 oils   Eicosapentaenoic Acid (EPA) $\rightarrow PGE_3$

$\downarrow$

Docosahexaenoic Acid (DHA)

Each member of the omega-3 and omega-6 families is used to make a specific prostaglandin. More importantly, these PGEs are used to make other, even more important, regulatory substances, such as thromboxanes and leukotrienes. Individually and collectively, they have profound effects on many body systems. For example, PGE_2 induces or antagonizes inflammation, and PGE_3 modulates it. Consequently, a diet rich in vegetables and fish will have the ability to balance inflammation because it will produce both PGE_2 and PGE_3. A diet richer in fish reduces inflammation because it will have more PGE_3. However, a diet devoid of fish, but with lots of meat, actually increases inflammation owing to the increased amounts of PGE_2. Therefore, people with rheumatoid arthritis should eat more fish. By eating more fish or taking EPA in supplement form, they can push their metabolism in the direction of more PGE_3. If they simultaneously eat to reduce PGE_2, they will favor the modulation of inflammation. We'll get to the prevention aspect soon.

The prostaglandins and their byproducts regulate many functions. These range from blood pressure and inflammation to the proliferation of some cancer cells, for example, breast cancer cells. Dyerberg found that breast cancer is nonexistent among the Greenlanders. Most experts think it's because other materials made from PGE_3, the leukotrienes, induce the Pac-Man cells and suppress certain cancer cells.

WHERE WE ARE AND WHERE WE'VE GOT TO GO

I've summarized the fat breakdown in the typical Western diet. In 1991, *Western* refers to North America, England, most of Europe, and the Scandinavian countries.

Salmon was once a staple in Scotland. Now all Scottish salmon is exported. Early in this century, Scottish apprentices went on strike against their employers because they were fed salmon. At the time, it was considered a garbage fish. The Scots eventually got away from fish eating and now have the highest rate of heart disease in the world and compete with England for the highest rate of inflammatory diseases. Some improvement!

TABLE 8.5

Fat Distribution in the American Diet

	Today	Longevity Diet
Percentage of total calories from fat	39 to 42	30 or less
Percentage of saturated fat	32 to 38	20
Percentage of monounsaturated fat	54 to 48	60
Percentage of polyunsaturated fat	14	20
Balance of polyunsaturated fat: Omega-6/Omega-3	3.2	1.0

Data extrapolated from various sources by the author including *The Journal of the American Dietetic Association, The Journal of the American College of Nutrition, The American Journal of Clinical Nutrition, The European Journal of Clinical Nutrition, The Journal of the Canadian Dietetic Association.*

Inspect the fat balance of omega-6 to omega-3 oils in table 8.5, because that's where you are today if you're average. It's not good, especially if you aren't a vigorous and regular exerciser. I've added a column that identifies the Longevity Diet, presented in chapter 15, which is where you want to be, especially in the balance of omega-6 to omega-3. The next thing you'll ask is: "Do I have to eat fish all the time?" No. All you've got to do is follow the Longevity Diet in chapter 15 and the guidelines at the end of this chapter.

FISH REALLY IS BRAIN FOOD: "THE REST OF THE STORY"

When scientists realized that DHA is necessary for the development of both eye and brain tissues, they did several experiments. First, studies in primates were conducted. Start the primates with a deficiency in DHA and their eye and brain tissues don't develop correctly. They don't see and learn as well as monkeys given enough DHA. Monkeys aren't people, but for experimental purposes they're as close as you can get, and they have only a

2-percent difference from us in their genes! The results of these studies told scientists what to look for in humans.

Case studies of DHA deficiency have begun to appear in the medical journals. There's no longer any question that DHA is essential for brain and eye development. Intuitively, you'd expect that to be the case because DHA is the most concentrated polyunsaturated fatty acid in both brain and eye tissues, especially the retina, and it wouldn't be so concentrated if it didn't serve an important purpose. When it's deficient in infancy or during development in the womb, these tissues don't develop correctly. Mental retardation and poor vision are the result. In view of what we know about selenium and Kaschin-Beck disease and vitamin C and childhood brain tumors, I wonder if predisposition to the inflammatory diseases doesn't also start in the womb? If it does, it would explain many findings that, at present, have no explanation. But that's for future research to unfold.

BREAST MILK AND DHA

Nature's wisdom is expressed in the components of breast milk. Why would breast milk concentrate selected food components at the mother's expense if they weren't essential for the developing infant? With the exception of some environmental chemicals, such as pesticides, also found there, breast milk contains exactly what the growing infant requires if the mother's diet is correct. DHA and EPA are found in breast milk. However, if the mother doesn't get either ALA or these oils in her food, they'll be missing in her milk.

DHA is required directly for growth and development while EPA is required for prevention of serious diseases. So when a mother elects to nurse her child, she's giving her infant the good start nature intended. Any woman who plans to have a child would be doing her child a favor by eating one serving of fish each day. The conditions necessary for proper child development start three months before conception and continue through to weaning from the breast. The Longevity Diet can take over after that.

WHAT ABOUT ADULT BRAIN FOOD?

Fish doesn't stop being brain food for infants and children; DHA is the most concentrated polyunsaturated fatty acid in the brain and eyes throughout life. Adults show a decline in vision when they don't get enough omega-3 oils. Specifically, the decline in vision parallels a decline of DHA in their eye tissue, especially in the retina.

What happens in the retina also takes place in the brain. We know DHA's loss costs sight in your eyes. Sight can be precisely measured, but what we don't know is what happens in our brain. We only know something must happen. I hope the future doesn't indicate that as DHA declines, it increases degenerative mental disorders that defy our present understanding.

HOW MUCH OMEGA-6 AND OMEGA-3 OILS?

Linoleic acid, the omega-6 oil that was designated by the Food and Nutrition Board as an essential fatty acid, is abundant in our diet. During the decades of the '50s, '60s, and '70s, scientists learned that a diet rich in polyunsaturated fats would help reduce cholesterol. This caused people to seek a convenient, inexpensive polyunsaturated oil; corn oil became king. As a result, we get much more omega-6, or linoleic acid, than the approximate two grams we need daily. In contrast, most people don't come close to the 1.2 or more grams of omega-3 oil experts conclude we need for optimum health. Indeed, it's likely that many people don't get close to the absolute minimum of three hundred milligrams of EPA daily. An adult should strive to get two grams of omega-3 oils daily.

Follow the Longevity Diet and you'll get enough omega-3 oil to meet your basic needs. Be sure to eat fish three times weekly and use the oils I've listed in table 8.6 in recipes and as a salad oil. We also add flaxseed oil to salad dressing. For frying, I recommend olive oil (a monounsaturated fat), or butter. Avoid using oils high in polyunsaturated fats for frying to reduce your risk of transforming polyunsaturated fats to the mildly toxic structure that many scientists believe promotes the risk of cancer. For baking cakes, breads, and other foods where oil is called for, the polyunsaturated oils are fine because the cooking temperatures are much lower. Better safe than sorry.

TABLE 8.6

Salad and Cooking Oils Rich in Omega-3

Oil	Percentage of Omega-6	Percentage of Omega-3
Menhaden	2	1
Soybean	51	7
Rapeseed	22	11
Canola	20	10
Salmon	22	10
Flaxseed	18	57

The remainder of the oils consist of monounsaturated and saturated oils.

WHICH FISH IS BEST?

"How do I know which fish to select?" Simple. The fish that comes from the coldest waters are best, as you can see in table 8.7. The fish from the coldest waters will require the most omega-3. Fish are poikilotherms, a big word that says they take on the temperature of their surroundings. So, the colder the water, the more omega-3 oils the fish need to keep from solidifying. Fish oil is still liquid at minus 103 degrees Fahrenheit!

Most omega-6 polyunsaturated fat is solid at cold ocean temperatures. I don't know if being cold makes these fish blue, but blue color (when they're viewed from the top) and omega-3 go together. Cold water, blue-skinned fish is about the best. Pink salmon flesh is a double protector because it contains both beta carotene and EPA. However, all fish, including seafood such as clams, oysters, lobsters, crabs, and squid, contain some omega-3 oil. You're always safe eating fish.

TABLE 8.7

The Best Fish to Eat

Fish	Omega-3 in grams	Fish	Omega-3 in grams
Sockeye salmon	3.0	Sardine	0.9
Albacore tuna	2.3	Whiting	0.9
Dogfish	2.0	Striped bass	0.7
Anchovy	1.9	Red snapper	0.6
Coho salmon	1.8	Freshwater catfish	0.6
Mackerel	1.8	King crab	0.6
Chinook salmon	1.7	Carp	0.5
Pink salmon	1.5	Shrimp	0.5
Freshwater trout	1.4	Ocean perch	0.4
American eel	1.3	Brook trout	0.4
Herring	1.3	Rockfish	0.3
Halibut	1.3	Sturgeon	0.2
Bluefin tuna	1.2	Haddock	0.2
Sablefish	1.2	Walleye	0.2
Swordfish	0.9	Cod	0.1
Mullet	0.9	Sole	0.1

All values are per 3½-ounce serving. Since 3½ ounces is also 100 grams, the amount of omega-3 is also the percentage of omega-3.

THERAPEUTIC USE OF FISH OIL SUPPLEMENTS

Hippocrates was the first physician to use an omega-3 oil therapeutically. His fifth-century use of flaxseed oil is consistent with twentieth-century science. Hippocrates observed that flaxseed oil, an excellent source of alpha linolenic acid, relieved inflammation of the mucous membranes of the bronchial tubes; we'd call it bronchial asthma. Hippocrates also used flaxseed oil for abdominal cramps associated with some types of diarrhea. This could be related to inflammatory bowel disease, but the information is too sketchy to tell.

Physicians are increasingly using fish oil in capsules as a therapeutic material. Actually flaxseed oil is almost as good as fish oil, is much cheaper, and can be used on food. EPA use in capsules, as an adjunct treatment for arthritis, psoriasis, inflammatory bowel disease, and other inflammatory diseases, is gaining acceptance. I've listed the omega-3 oil content of some supplements in table 8.8.

TABLE 8.8

Omega-3 Oil Supplements

Supplement		Mg Per Capsule
Shaklee EPA		325
Max EPA		325
Super EPA		360
Codliver oil, per teaspoon	1.72 grams	
Flaxseed oil, per teaspoon	2.60 grams	

Angioplasty is a medical procedure used for clearing an artery clogged with plaque. The operation is done by inserting, through a large vein, a special balloon that, when inflated, compresses the plaque and opens the artery. Twenty-five to 35 percent of people who have angioplasty to open clogged arteries develop reclogging within six months. Taking a daily supplement of 3 to 6 grams of omega-3 oils reduces the reclogging by about 60 percent. However, more research is underway to quantify both the amount of omega-3 oil necessary and the effect produced.

EPA supplements are increasingly being used in the management of multiple sclerosis. Dermatologists are also using EPA to reduce attacks of psoriasis and scleroderma.

Arthritis is significantly improved by taking 15 capsules containing a total of 2.5 grams of EPA and 1.8 grams of DHA daily. The oils in the capsules are somewhat diluted, so it was necessary to take 15 of them to get the required amount. It's unrealistic for the average person, but in clinical research it proved the point. A study of this regimen, conducted by Dr. Joel M. Kremer and his colleagues at the Albany Medical School, gave results found to be typical. In fourteen weeks, or three and a half months, every arthritis symptom, such as tenderness of joints, swelling, grip strength, and stiffness, had improved by 50 percent or more. Compared to the side effects of drugs, even those of aspirin, which is normally used for arthritis, the side effects of EPA consist of nothing more than a fishy taste and bad breath and are completely insignificant medically.

Several papers have been published showing that the omega-3 oils help relieve ulcerative colitis, an inflammatory bowel disease. Leukotrienes, metabolic products from PGE_3, are the actual agents that reduce the ulcerative colitis flare-up. This finding has opened a new approach to the treatment of inflammatory bowel diseases. We owe a lot to Dyerberg's persistent studies.

ANECDOTAL SUPPORT FROM WORLD WAR II

During a tour of England to promote my book *The Arthritis Relief Diet*, which appeared in the United Kingdom as *Arthritis: Diet Against It*, I encountered an unexpected observation. My book explains a dietary approach for people with inflammatory disease. It teaches how to use fish and fish oils in a dietary plan to enhance medical support for arthritis. When people heard me talk, they often commented that during the war their parents' arthritis cleared up. It was fish oil again, but this time with some unplanned, government help.

In World War II, all children in England were provided with a daily cod liver oil supplement to be sure they got sufficient vitamin A and D; adults took it as well. Even though it tastes terrible, people learned to accept it. A tablespoon of cod liver oil provides one gram of EPA and half a gram of DHA. Add this to the low-fat wartime diet, and an excellent balance of omega-6 oils to omega-3 oils was achieved. No one intended for the cod liver oil supplement to be a nutritional experiment, so no records were kept. However, it worked so well that, in 1989, fifty years later, people were still talking about how their parents' arthritis had cleared up.

IS MORE BETTER? SAFETY?

Thanks to modern technology, we can purchase omega-3 oil supplements easily. This convenience means that there's no reason not to get enough. But it also raises the specter of too much.

Some confusion seems to prevail about the upper limit to omega-3 oils. My review of the safety literature leads me to believe that most people who follow the Longevity Diet don't need to take more than three capsules, or about one gram of fish oil daily. If you're following a dietary plan for arthritis, twice as much, or six capsules, should be enough.

In many clinical studies, up to twenty-five capsules, or over eight grams daily were used with no adverse side effects. However, 8 or more grams of EPA from supplements can lengthen blood-clotting time. Longer clotting time indicates that people who are on heart attack or stroke medication could create a modest health risk with such high levels of fish-oil supplements. These people should consult with their physician before taking more than 2 grams of fish oil daily.

WHAT CAN YOU DO?

Although I've emphasized both omega-6 and omega-3 oils, your diet will provide more than enough omega-6 no matter how you eat. People in the United States don't get enough omega-3 oils. A few steps will make sure you get all you need.

- Eat 3 servings of fish weekly; 4 servings or more are even better. Don't eat or count deep-fat-fried "square" fish from fast food outlets; they have no omega-3 oils. Use table 8.7 as a guide for fish selection.

- Use omega-3 oils, such as canola oil, in salads and in baking, whenever possible. Let table 8.6 be your guide. Though these oils cost more, look at them as an insurance policy. Add flaxseed oil to your salad oil; it's tasteless and imparts a nice golden hue.

- Omega-3 oil supplements are fine. Strive for 500 milligrams of omega-3 oils as supplements each day if you don't eat fish. These oils should list the amount of EPA and DHA on the nutritional label.

- Don't fry with corn oil or oil high in polyunsaturated fats. Always use olive oil, if possible, and peanut oil or even butter as a last resort.

- Snack on nuts that grow on trees. Peanuts are goobers that grow in the ground, and they don't contain omega-3 oils.

WHAT DO I DO?

At home I eat fish four or more times weekly and add a teaspoon of flaxseed oil to my food each day. When I travel and my diet suffers, I take 500 milligrams of omega-3 oils daily as a supplement.

9

Gamma Linolenic Acid

In 1621, friendly Indians taught the Pilgrims to use oil from the seeds of the evening primrose plant as medicine. The Indians used this oil as an anti-inflammatory, probably for premenstrual cramps, and as a general analgesic. Anthropologists have found that most American Indians had some osteoarthritis, so the oil's anti-inflammatory properties were probably very helpful. The Pilgrims were so impressed by its curative properties that they sent the plant back to England, where the plant was cultivated, and the oil became known as the "king's cure-all."

The "cure-all" concept of evening primrose oil was widely accepted up to the twentieth century. *American Medical Plants,* published in 1892, describes the evening primrose as a plant of important therapeutic value for inflammatory disorders. The text goes on to explain the significance of the oil.

Gamma Linolenic Acid Quiz

- Do you or someone you know regularly get premenstrual stress?

173

- Have you or anyone you know been diagnosed as a manic depressive or as being schizophrenic?

- Do you or someone you know regularly use nonsteroid, anti-inflammatory drugs?

- Do you or anyone you know have Raynaud's syndrome?

If you answered yes to any one of the above questions, you will benefit from learning more about gamma linolenic acid.

Seeds of evening primrose contain several important nutrients, including linoleic acid, gamma linolenic acid (GLA), and vitamin E. GLA is an omega-6 oil that the body converts to the prostaglandin, PGE_1.

The Omega-6 Oils Family

Internal Metabolism

Food Source	Food Acid	Prostaglandins
Vegetable oils and animal flesh	Linoleic Acid	
	↓	
No normal, dietary source: Evening primrose seed oil Black currant seed oil Borage Oil	GLA	
	↓	
	Extended GLA →	PGE_1
	↓	
Animal fat and animal products	Arachidonic Acid →	PGE_2

Normally we would expect linoleic acid to be converted to GLA for making all of the prostaglandin PGE_1 that the body needs. After all, GLA is readily made from linoleic acid, and with all the vegetable oils entering the food system, we get plenty, if not an excess, of linoleic acid. However, some scientists point out that certain people and some dietary circumstances don't allow enough linoleic acid to be made into GLA; consequently, there's a deficiency of the prostaglandin. I'll return to the reasoning behind this in a moment.

We have an abundance of arachidonic acid (AA) and its prostaglandin PGE_2 because we get plenty of AA from the flesh of animals, birds, fish, and the animal fat in dairy products. Indeed, some experts suggest that we get too much arachidonic acid. So it would seem we're dealing with a unique situation when there's a GLA shortfall. Some scientists are skeptical about the importance of GLA, even though the oil of evening primrose has stood a 250-year test of time that we know of.

A hypothesis suggests that there are two interrelated circumstances that favor insufficient PGE_1. Some people lack the ability to make GLA in sufficient quantity to supply enough PGE_1 when it's needed. Secondary to this is our diet, so rich in the other two omega-6 oils that our metabolic system can become swamped, and GLA production is simply obliterated by a process called "mass action."

There are several circumstances that favor this hypothesis. It suggests that GLA might be needed as a therapeutic supplement for some, and possibly many, people. Two areas of support for GLA will help you see why the subject of GLA is left open for discussion and investigation.

CAN MOTHER'S MILK BE WRONG?

Human mother's milk is the best, if not the only, dietary source of GLA. Would it be in mother's milk if there wasn't a need? I don't believe it would, because it takes energy to make GLA, like other nutrients, such as taurine, that we find in mother's milk. Experience teaches us that every nutrient scientists discover in mother's milk is essential for the growing infant. The same nutrient is usually required by adults as well.

Prostaglandin PGE_1 made from GLA is involved in immune function. Although we can't say that the immune system doesn't develop as well without GLA, there is good scientific evidence to support this theory. There's proof that breastfed children have a better immune system not only during nursing, but also six months after weaning, compared to children who were formula fed. The only chemical difference between the infant formula tested and breast milk is GLA. Even though this immune difference is not conclusive evidence and calls for more research, it's consistent with the concept that GLA wouldn't be in mother's milk if it wasn't necessary.

PREMENSTRUAL SYNDROME (PMS)

At the EFAMOL Research Institute, Dr. David Horrobin developed the hypothesis of a marginal deficiency of GLA in PMS. He based his idea on some indirect data that suggested some women couldn't make enough GLA from linoleic acid to satisfy their needs. Horrobin theorizes that inadequate GLA produces a shortage of PGE_1. In women, a shortage of PGE_1 produces a spectrum of symptoms we call premenstrual syndrome (PMS).

PMS symptoms include depression, irritability, breast pain and tenderness, and fluid retention, beginning three to ten days before the monthly period. To test Horrobin's hypothesis, a number of female volunteers were divided into two groups; one group was given from 180 to 360 milligrams of GLA daily and the other group was given a placebo.

It worked! After three months, 50 percent of the women who got GLA had moderate to complete relief of PMS symptoms, compared to 6 percent of the placebo controls. Other studies produced results ranging from 30- to 70-percent effectiveness, depending on the level of GLA taken and the time of use. Since the placebo produced a 6- to 10-percent reduction in every PMS study, we can safely conclude the studies were valid. The only issue left open is how effective GLA is. Since PMS symptoms are not precise, the results should be expected to vary widely among women.

Secondary support for Horrobin's hypothesis was derived from the blood analysis of women with PMS. All women with PMS have unusually high levels of linoleic acid, which suggests that their linoleic acid wasn't being converted to GLA. Horrobin further hypothesized that PMS sufferers were unable to make enough GLA because of a hereditary deficiency.

Horrobin's hypothesis is very specific, right down to the enzyme that converts linoleic acid to GLA. Therefore, this enzyme shortage is another biochemical line of support for his theory.

A DIETARY DILEMMA

Horrobin's success with PMS has created a dilemma. How often does your diet include seeds of the evening primrose or black currant? That's the point: GLA is a substance most diets only provide in trace amounts.

A reasonable amount of searching leads me to conclude that the Northeastern American Indians, who introduced the evening primrose oil, didn't eat the seeds of evening primrose either. You'd have to eat a lot of black currants to get the 180 milligrams of GLA used in the studies, so why bother with Horrobin's ideas at all?

Horrobin's hypothesis has gained support from many scientific groups. He believes that our ability to make GLA diminishes as a result of dietary excesses that interfere with the body's natural enzymes that make GLA from linoleic acid. GLA was once a nutrient that we only needed as infants, but now that we've elected to eat and live as we do, it's also needed by many adults. Some of the dietary excesses that create the need for GLA in adults are as follows:

- Eating a lot of saturated fats. Saturated fat interferes with the availability of linoleic acid. In short, it blocks linoleic acid. So a diet high in saturated fat—the typical American diet— would result in a GLA deficiency.

- Eating a high-fat diet. The abundance of arachidonic acid (AA) in our diet causes "feedback inhibition." Think of this inhibition as a traffic jam on a bridge that backs up traffic. You might not need to cross the bridge, but if you're in the jam, it doesn't matter. You still don't move. Imagine an abundance of AA in your tissues from our generally high-fat diet. Now think of this abundance as a signal that says: "I'm full." Since our metabolic system is not designed for this AA abundance, this signal causes a slowdown of everything, including GLA production. That's how feedback inhibition works—the end product acts as a roadblock for the entire process.

- Eating cooked foods high in linoleic acid. In nature, linoleic acid exists in a form that is changed by processing and frying. The natural form is called "cis" and the other is called "trans." Cis-linoleic acid is converted to equal amounts of cis and trans by processing. Though both forms can be used for energy, it appears that both can't be made into GLA, only the cis form. When trans is present, it poisons the process that makes GLA. It's as if someone tied your hands and jaw, making it very difficult for you to eat. So even though there was an abundance of food available, you'd lose weight.

- Eating a high-sugar diet, coupled with being seriously over-weight. This combination produces a prediabetic condition in 10 to 20 percent of adults. This prediabetes causes an impairment in our ability to make GLA, even if we are not yet to the point where treatment for the diabetes is necessary.

There are also conditions not related to dietary excess that cause insufficient GLA, including marginal zinc deficiency, virus infections, and aging.

According to the hypothesis, our rich diet and general over-weight reduce the production of GLA. And some people, such as PMS sufferers, for example, are unable to make enough GLA because of a hereditary deficiency.

CLINICAL HORIZONS

GLA is the subject of many intensive investigations. I counted over one hundred and fifty-five studies begun between 1987 and 1990. The number of these studies will escalate and they will continue into the next century if the preliminary results on GLA continue to be reinforced. Here are the areas in which GLA research is proving most intriguing.

- *Schizophrenia:* Levels of PGE_1 are deficient compared to PGE_2 and PGE_3 in schizophrenics, so the use of evening primrose oil was tested for a positive effect. Even though the results with evening primrose oil were disappointing, the use of specific PGE_1 promoters was effective, so the research is continuing. These preliminary findings suggest that there's an effect taking place in schizophrenics involving GLA or PGE_1 that deserves more research.

- *Manic depression:* This mental disorder is characterized by excessive PGE_1 in the manic phase and not enough in the depression phase. Drugs used to control manic depression block PGE_1 production. Scientists are seriously studying ways to achieve the same effect with GLA or a combination of GLA and drugs.

- *Attention deficit disorder:* This disorder is more commonly known as hyperactivity in children. Hyperactive children treated with supplemental GLA have shown definite improvement. These early findings suggest that hyperactivity results from, among other things, an imbalance of the essential oils or prostaglandin production.

- *Autoimmune diseases:* Some autoimmune diseases, such as rheumatoid arthritis, atopic eczema, and multiple sclerosis, have improved with supplemental GLA. The most encouraging result indicates that GLA can replace nonsteroid antiinflammatory drugs in many people. Since GLA has no known side-effects, its use is favored over the drugs.

- *Neuropathy:* In these conditions, nerves do not conduct impulses correctly and become nonfunctional. An area of the body affected will tingle and become so insensitive that it can be poked with a needle and feel no pain. GLA reduces symptoms in 75 percent of the variables tested. These results are being very actively pursued.

- *Raynaud's syndrome:* This form of arthritis creates a special cold sensitivity and is characterized by arthritislike attacks. In a double-blind study, GLA effectively reduced flare-ups of this disease.

- *Sjogren's Syndrome:* This disease is characterized by the lack of tear production. It is caused by an inability to make GLA and is completely relieved by GLA supplements.

IS GLA A NUTRIENT? IS IT A DRUG?

GLA wouldn't be abundant in mother's milk if it didn't serve a nutritional purpose. When it is used to relieve symptoms—even something as non-life-threatening as PMS—according to lawmakers, it becomes a drug. But it is a dietary factor anyone can get from the evening primrose plant. It has no side effects that characterize even the mildest drug, such as baby aspirin.

Are we witnessing the recognition that some people have unusual nutrient requirements because of our modern lifestyle? Does this mean that in the future some people will take a daily supplement of GLA? If they do, will GLA be seen as a nutrient their diet simply can't provide? Or will it be a drug?

10

Folic Acid

Monkeys, chicks, some bacteria, and humans require a growth factor that is found in vegetables, especially spinach and other leafy green vegetables. This foliage factor is easily destroyed by cooking and so remained elusive until 1943, when it was finally isolated from spinach leaves. Folacin seemed like the most appropriate name for this new vitamin in recognition of its main source, the foliage of green, leafy vegetables.

Folacin is a storage form of folic acid. As an acid, folacin is combined with other materials in the plant, and our body activates all these combined forms into folic acid. The only available source of free folic acid are milk and food supplements.

Folic acid is one of seven B vitamins. It is actually a synthesis of three natural chemicals: pteridine, which gives the yellow, phosphorescent color to butterfly wings; para-aminobenzoic acid, an acid common in plants that we excrete when we eat cranberries; and glutamic acid, an amino acid found in most proteins. So technically it's pteroylglutamic acid. Most plants make folic acid readily from its three components, but most animals, including humans, can't make it at all. We absolutely require folic acid for life.

Folic Acid Quiz

Answer yes or no to the following questions:

- Do you take medication, including birth control pills, regularly?

- Has a birth defect, such as a cleft palate, hairlip, or spina bifida, ever occurred in your family?

- Have you or a blood relative ever been anemic or had long periods of chronic fatigue?

- Do you have frequent diarrhea or very loose stools?

A yes answer to any question suggests that you should learn more about folic acid.

WHAT POPEYE KNEW

During the cartoon heyday of the 1940s, Popeye the Sailorman became known to children of all ages. If you remember Popeye, you remember his love, Olive Oyl, and his archrival, Bluto. Olive was forever being chased and abducted by Bluto. She'd holler to Popeye for help, but he was often fatigued, weak, and sleepy; in short, he was unequal to the task until he ate a can of spinach. "I'm strong to the finish, cause I eats my spinach," he'd sing after subduing Bluto and rescuing Olive. Popeye's symptoms of weakness and fatigue were graphic examples of folic acid deficiency; the cartoonist left out headaches.

Popeye was a modern version of a long line of mythical figures, going back over one thousand years, that were used to get children and even adults to eat foods that are good for them. Usually the foods chosen were green vegetables, the ones children often avoid. Even though these myths promoted foods with many important nutrients, one nutrient common to all was folic acid.

Folic acid is essential in order for the body to manufacture the building blocks of our genetic material. It is also essential in making several amino acids, the building blocks of protein. The breakdown and use by the body of some amino acids also require folic acid. If you get the impression that folic acid is important in cell reproduction, you're correct. In fact, cell reproduction can't take place correctly when there's not enough folic acid, nor can the body build protein. In summary, folic acid is critical in cell division and for protein manufacture.

Folic acid's requirement in cell division goes even one step further. Folic acid is a helper in an enzyme system that corrects defects in DNA, the most basic genetic material. This gives it a second purpose in cell reproduction.

An important part of protein synthesis is the manufacture of antibodies. These proteins are the materials that actually attack viruses and other things to which we've become immune. Since folic acid is essential in their production, it is an indirect but important part of the immune system.

FOLIC ACID DEFICIENCY

Folic acid deficiency is usually described by nutritionists by its symptoms: a smooth, red tongue; intestinal upset and diarrhea; along with fatigue, weakness, and headaches. However, the primary problem is an anemia (macrocytic anemia) in which there are fewer red blood cells. The red blood cells that exist are larger in size and contain less of the oxygen-carrying pigment hemoglobin. "Macro" means large, and "cytic" means cells.

This basic anemia explained the gross symptoms. Red blood cells carry oxygen, and if there are not enough red blood cells or they don't function correctly, all the symptoms of oxygen starvation will prevail. Not enough oxygen to the brain and muscles will result in headaches, fatigue, weakness, and even confusion. Sound like Popeye's symptoms?

But scientists knew there should be more to this anemia. Red blood cells are always being produced, so there shouldn't be a shortage of them. And the cells being produced are not normal. An inspection of red blood cells in bone marrow, where they're produced, showed lots of immature and abnormal cells. In short, production of blood cells had stopped in the wrong place; in a sense, production was not completed. In order to see more clearly what was causing these effects, why not look at periods of more critical requirements for cell reproduction, like pregnancy? During the first three months of pregnancy, a woman's body is called on to make an enormous amount of new tissue. Indeed, she becomes a biological factory. So if any nutrient deficiencies have an affect during this early phase of pregnancy, their effects should stand in bold relief.

It didn't take long for scientists to create folic acid deficiencies in experimental animals during early pregnancy. Sure enough, cleft lip, skeletal deformities, and eye defects were observed, in addition to fluid retention in the skull and spine. The logical question arose: Could this happen to people?

FOLIC ACID AS A PROTECTOR

In 1965 the English medical journal *The Lancet* carried a paper entitled "Folic Acid Metabolism and Human Embryopathy," by Drs. E. D. Hibbard and R. W. Smithells. They suggested a relationship between certain malformations of the fetal central nervous system, called neural tube defects, and defective folic acid metabolism. Shortly after that, Smithells reported two women who delivered children with neural tube defects. Both women had been on anticonvulsant drugs that interfere with folic acid metabolism.

During the third or fourth week of pregnancy the infant is still an embryo with an open, tubelike structure called the neural tube. This tube will form the brain, spinal cord, and the spinal column of the baby after it closes; so it's often complete before a woman even knows she's pregnant. At the time of the *Lancet* report, it was common practice for a woman to wait until she missed two menstrual cycles before being considered pregnant. If folic acid was short, it was too late by then to make up for the deficit.

If this neural tube fails to close correctly at the base of the spine, spina bifida develops. The effects of spina bifida can range from the appearance of a dimple at the base of the child's spine with no serious consequences to a severe defect in which the spine actually protrudes through the back. In these severe cases, the child will have serious, completely debilitating defects and is usually profoundly crippled.

If the neural tube fails to close at the top, the brain doesn't develop correctly and may even be completely missing. This situation almost always results in the death of the fetus or the death of the child shortly after birth. If the child survives, it is always severely retarded.

The risk of neural tube defects among North American women is low in the absence of a family history of them. There's about a 2-percent risk if there's a family history of the defect. Risk of neural tube defects is lower among blacks than whites. The risk is higher in England and Ireland than in North America. Though 2 percent doesn't sound high, it's the second leading cause of death among infants who die from birth defects.

Since Hibbard and Smithells published their paper, many studies have been conducted in the United States, Britain, Ireland, and Australia with similar and consistent results. At least six major studies are still underway in the United States, Britain, Egypt, and Ireland. The object of these current studies is to fully understand how this defect occurs. Experts know it's related to folic acid and its effect on cell reproduction; it's just that they don't understand why it occurs in some women and not others. It's most likely to strike in women who have already had one child with a neural tube defect.

In one typical study in Ireland, seven hundred and forty-four women were selected who had had one child with a neural tube defect. Half the women were supplemented with folic acid and half were given a placebo before and during their next pregnancy. Only four children with neural tube defects were born to the women who got supplements. There were sixteen among the unsupplemented women. A 75-percent reduction of a serious defect from about five cents' worth of a vitamin is an astronomical return on an investment.

CLEFT LIP: CLEFT PALATE

Clefts of the lip or palate, the roof of the mouth, occur once in about seven hundred and fifty births. The severity of this defect varies widely and can be corrected by cosmetic surgery. In minor cases, it can be corrected within the first year. In severe cases, corrective surgery requires many operations, often up to the age of eighteen. Sometimes another operation is required after age twenty-one to "tidy things" left by the other operations.

Low levels of folic acid and smoking during pregnancy have been associated with these defects. These defects also seem to occur in families, and women who have delivered one child with the defect are likely to deliver another.

Three major research studies were conducted on women who had already had a child with a cleft defect. A comparison of one group of these women who were given supplemental folic acid with another group who didn't get folic acid showed striking results. Over 4 percent of the women who didn't take folic acid delivered a second child with the cleft defect. In contrast, only 1 percent of women who took folic acid delivered a second, defective child— small investment; large return.

DOES FORM EQUAL FUNCTION?

All research has produced similar results. Folic acid supplements, begun as early as possible in pregnancy, reduce both neural tube and cleft birth defects dramatically. After one large Australian study was published, the journal editors raised the question: Does the form of folic acid make a difference?

These studies suggest that the folic acid deficiency in some women may be the result of a lack of the ability to activate some dietary forms of folic acid and not a result of insufficient dietary folic acid. In supplements, folic acid is in its free form—we call it "unconjugated"—therefore, it doesn't need to be activated.

If this hypothesis can be proven, it would explain why these defects aren't more widespread. But more importantly, the hypothesis provides a research approach that could lead to their complete elimination.

CANCER: THEORY

Neural tube defect studies prove that if there isn't enough folic acid at critical times in development, serious consequences can result. Drawing this conclusion requires a great deal of knowledge and is a major step up from just recognizing the small, weak red blood cells of common folic acid deficiency. It didn't take long for the theoretical biologist to follow the thread of cell development and propose other, more serious consequences of folic acid deficiency.

Theorists reasoned that dysplastic cells should be observed in folic acid deficiency. After all, when a cell can't divide correctly, it's a form of dysplasia. Though red blood cells are simple, uncomplicated cells compared to cells of the intestines or uterus, in folic acid deficiency, the red blood cells aren't normal. They're larger than normal and have less hemoglobin. That's dysplasia, albeit a minor form.

The red blood cell doesn't reproduce like other cells; it's manufactured in the bone marrow; it doesn't split to reproduce itself. So if it's a dysplastic cell, it doesn't matter as far as reproduction is concerned. But the concept has serious consequences in cells that do reproduce.

FOLIC ACID PREVENTS DYSPLASIA

Carry dysplasia one more step in cells that reproduce, and you've got the chance of developing cancer. After all, dysplastic cells are known precursors to cancer in tissues such as the mouth, intestines, uterus, and the bladder. Dysplasia is probably involved in other tissues as well, so the theorist sees a relationship between folic acid and cancer that starts with dysplasia.

Three studies tested the hypothesis that supplemental folic acid would reduce dysplasia. All three supported the hypothesis. Theory and practice came to the same point. This conclusion gave scientists cause to reinterpret data from the 1950s, when folic acid had only been known for seven years as a nutrient. In those days, pathologists followed people who got anemia from folic acid deficiency, because they were more likely to get gastric cancer. This result now gave them cause to connect the cancer to folic acid deficiency.

Dysplasia was also observed in the uterus of women with folic acid deficiency. Then it was seen again in some women on the birth control pill, which we'll discuss shortly.

Other researchers observed that folic acid would reverse dysplastic cells that occurred in the bronchial tubes of smokers. Another tissue became involved; supplemental folic acid made dysplastic cells return to normal. In this case, the smoking caused dysplasia, and it increased the need for folic acid.

CANCER WITH A BAD GUT

People who have inflammatory bowel disease (IBD), such as ulcerative colitis, colitis, ileitis, or Crohn's disease, are twenty-five times more likely than normal folks to get cancer. In fact, about 13 percent of people with these diseases die of colon cancer; that's far above the national average. Since many other sufferers of IBD have their colon removed entirely, this is an astronomical rate of colon cancer.

People with these diseases have two strikes against them. First strike: the disease is characterized by poor folic acid absorption from their food. Second strike: the drug used to treat most of them, sulfasalazine, interferes with folic acid absorption. People with these diseases are the ideal group to compare cancer rates in people who take folic acid supplements and people who don't.

Colonic cancer among people with IBD is 50 percent less if they take folic acid supplements! This finding correlates very well with an older observation, that people with a bad gut have blood levels of folic acid about 50 percent of normal. So theory and reality come together again.

Women on the birth control pill, people taking sulfasalazine, and smokers raise a question: Do these people experience a localized deficiency of folic acid? Could the hormonal changes brought on by the pill cause the uterus tissues to be deficient in folic acid even if blood levels of folic acid are low but within normal limits? Would the same situation hold true for sulfasalazine and the colonic tissues, or smoking and the bronchial membranes? These questions are critical because they collide with the issue of how much folic acid we need.

Animal studies have answered these questions. They confirm that folic acid deficiency can be localized and increases the likelihood of dysplasia. However, they also confirm that these dysplastic cells don't become cancerous unless a cancer initiator is present; for instance, a nitrosamine, a pesticide, or a circumstance that causes free radicals to develop. An example would be a chlorinated hydrocarbon in drinking water that becomes a chlorine superoxide in the body, or exposure to noxious fumes.

DYSPLASIA: A DEFICIENCY DISEASE?

A dysplased or dysplastic cell is one that's somewhere between a normal and a cancerous cell. A cell can become dysplased by an irritant, such as the materials in tobacco or betel nuts, to name two. But the results with folic acid suggest something much more profound: Cells can become dysplased from a shortage of folic acid! It raises an important question: Is dysplasia a deficiency disease?

If folic acid shortfall increases the likelihood of dysplastic cells developing, where does that place the average person? Many things besides diet cause folic acid to become short. Most common shortfalls are produced by drugs. Some of the drugs that cause a deficiency in folic acid are:

- Birth control pills
- Aspirin
- Azulfidine
- Methotrexate
- Cholesterol-lowering medication

- Antacids
- Anticonvulsant medication
- Anti-inflammatory drugs
- Gold shots
- Diuretics

Other causes of folic acid shortfalls, when a person gets a good diet, are obscure. I can explain this through a clinical study in which I was involved.

We put a large group of college women on a balanced diet to test the effectiveness of a supplement program. After four weeks on the balanced diet, blood samples were analyzed for selected vitamins and minerals; one of them was folic acid. Folic acid was the only vitamin that was near the bottom of the normal range in about 10 percent of the women. It was easily brought to the middle range with either dietary adjustment or a supplement.

Why did these women have such low levels of folic acid? They had no symptoms of deficiency. All were healthy as determined by the physicians monitoring the program. Some used birth control pills; others didn't. In short, these women probably didn't absorb or handle folic acid as well as the rest. But how do you know if you're like one of these college women?

HOW MUCH DO WE NEED?

Folic acid was a problem one thousand years ago and also in 1980 when the RDA was four hundred micrograms for average people. In 1989, the RDA was lowered by 50 percent to two hundred micrograms. Before 1989, just about every food survey conducted showed that over 70 percent of the population often fell below 50 percent of the RDA for folic acid. Folic acid deficiency is still one of the most widespread nutrient deficiencies worldwide. In spite of our RDA, there are even deficiencies in America.

Before 1989, most nutrition texts stated it as Hamilton and Whitney did on page 274 in the second edition, 1982, of *Nutrition: Concepts and Controversies,* a widely used text: "Not only is folacin deficiency the most common vitamin deficiency in people, it is also most likely to be caused by the taking of medication."

The RDA committee recognized how much folic acid is generally in the food supply and that there are no deficiency symptoms. However, the committee also pointed out that megoblastic anemia is the late-stage symptom of deficiency; it's like scurvy and vitamin C deficiency. They also took into account body reservoirs and made a conservative estimate that only 50 percent is absorbed from food.

The committee didn't include the following issues when determining the RDA for folic acid: presence of dysplastic cells, susceptibility to cancer, and family history of birth defects. Are these the tip of a bigger iceberg?

Even though cancer and birth defects have always been serious concerns, we're just now coming to grips with the nutrition issues. We recognize that excess fat and excess calories are involved, but the notion that a marginal nutritional deficiency is involved is very difficult to deal with: it's like trying to nail Jell-O to a tree!

FOLIC ACID FROM FOOD

We're back to the old concept of a balanced diet. Who eats one? The Longevity Diet will provide the RDA for folic acid. It's worthwhile to review the foods that supply folic acid. I've done this in table 10.1.

TABLE 10.1

Folic Acid in Food

Food Source	Folic Acid, in Micrograms
Asparagus	116
Beet greens	50
Beans, various	90
Broccoflower	92
Broccoli	54
Brussels sprouts	80
Peas, average	130
Corn	50
Cranberry beans	180
Okra	134
Parsley	55
Seaweed	180
Spinach	130
Liver	250
Yeast, average per ounce	575
Cereals, if fortified	100

All servings are ½ cup except liver, which is 3½ ounces of beef, pork, or lamb liver. Other vegetables and fruits provide 15 to 25 micrograms of folic acid per serving.

By inspecting table 10.1, you can see that deep green vegetables and beans are the best sources of folic acid. The Longevity Diet exceeds the 1989 RDA of folic acid and will even meet the 1980 RDA.

Excessive cooking can destroy folic acid. Steam vegetables and learn to enjoy them when they're crisp. Eat peas and beans regularly and when selecting a high-fiber cereal, read the nutrition label to be sure it contains about 100 micrograms of folic acid.

DO YOU NEED SUPPLEMENTS?

I can't answer this question for you, but you can decide for yourself. Consider the following questions:

- Do you regularly use medication? For example:
  Birth control pills
  Analgesics, such as aspirin
  Anti-inflammatory medication
  Anticonvulsant medication
  Tranquilizers
  Cholesterol-lowering drugs
  High blood pressure medication
  Intestinal medication

- Are you planning to become pregnant within the next six months?

- Do you have difficulty gaining weight?

- Do you have frequent diarrhea?

If you answered yes to any of these questions, you should take a multivitamin-multimineral supplement daily that provides at least 100 micrograms of folic acid. It's a very cheap insurance policy.

SAFETY

Folic acid is one of the seven B vitamins. When taken in excess of up to ten times the RDA, it is safe. At levels of one hundred times the RDA, problems sometimes develop. However, over twenty times the 1989 RDA is in the range where folic acid is considered a physiologically active chemical; some experts say "drug levels." Levels that high are definitely not the domain of nutritionists.

PRECONCEPTION NUTRITION

Birth defects I've described here are serious. They occur in the first four weeks of pregnancy. No one has any idea of what role marginal deficiencies have in minor birth defects. Indeed, in variations we'd still call normal, there are probably many.

However, the first four weeks of pregnancy often pass before you know you're pregnant. Worse yet, suppose you just went off the pill and have low folic-acid levels. The doctor is likely to say,

"See me when you've missed two periods"; that's eight weeks. Adding folic acid after that is necessary, but it can be like closing the door after the horse has escaped. That's why the concept of preconception nutrition is so important.

If you're thinking of having a baby, take preconception nutrition seriously. A multivitamin-multimineral supplement with up to 400 micrograms of folic acid costs about ten cents a day. In a society of people who spend sixty cents per day per capita on soft drinks and subsidize tobacco smoking and chewing, ten cents spent for nutrition would be a bargain at five times the price.

GET ENOUGH FOLIC ACID

Stick to the Longevity Diet; it calls for:

- Five servings of green vegetables and fruit daily
- Whole grain cereal daily
- Whole grain bread daily
- Beans once daily

11

Niacin

Mead, an alcoholic beverage with a golden hue, was the nectar of the gods in ancient Greece. It was made by fermenting honey. A thousand years later, in the middle ages, it was the beverage of feudal lords. Though its alcohol made people feel important, livened conversation, and helped the world look better, mead was also a nutritional bonus.

Honey is about 99 percent simple sugars, called glucose and fructose, with some water. Honey has no significant nutritional value besides calories. But ferment the honey, or any sugar for that matter, and you're raising yeast—strange to think of brewing as "yeast farming," but that's one way to look at it. Yeast, in contrast to the sugar on which it's grown, is a nutritional powerhouse. It contains protein, minerals from the water, and vitamins, including the all important B vitamins, especially niacin.

Yeast saved from the fermentation of honey has been fed to infants and children throughout history and worked its way into a variety of foods. Yeast was probably the single most nourishing food, after mother's milk, that was readily available to children all year round. Beers made the old-fashioned way and not refrigerated are similarly nourishing. Yeast also became a significant part of old-fashioned bread that was heavy by our standards but very nour-

194

ishing. In fact, bread was so nourishing it became the first request in the Lord's Prayer.

Chapter 10 showed us how a deficiency of one of the B vitamins, folic acid, can cause dysplastic cells and birth defects. Another member of the vitamin B team, niacin, has a history as colorful as folic acid's, and we are now recognizing it as the most fundamental of all protectors. You could say its protection was designed by God. But first we'll consider niacin the nutrient, and then segue into its marvelous protector function.

Niacin Quiz

Answer yes or no to the following questions:

- Do you think that the term *redneck* describes people who are inherently stupid and lazy?

- Do you think honey is a nourishing food?

- Can mistakes in DNA (genetic material) occur at random and cause cancer?

If you answered yes to any of these questions, you can learn much about an important protector by reading this chapter.

PELLAGRA AND REDNECKS

In 1915, over two hundred thousand people living in the southern part of the United States came down with pellagra. Pellagra is derived from the Italian words, *pelle,* meaning skin, and *agara,* meaning rough. Once established, pellagra is characterized by red, rough skin. The first physical symptom of niacin deficiency is red skin that is very sensitive to sunlight. So the first people affected by niacin deficiency were farmworkers whose exposed faces, hands, and necks became red and sore. But even before the skin sensitivity appears, a deficiency of niacin causes mental dullness and depression. Therefore, it didn't take long for people to label people with red necks as slow and dull.

Niacin and some other B vitamin deficiencies are called the "three Ds," which stand for *dementia, dermatitis,* and *diarrhea,* the symptoms that appear in that order. In 1915, the first symptom seen was dermatitis—red skin. In fact, many people who were cured of the physical symptoms spent the remainder of their lives in mental institutions because their mental decline had passed the point of being cured by restoring the vitamin.

In 1915, about ten thousand of these Southerners died from the deficiency of niacin and over two hundred thousand were seriously affected. It all happened because they lacked a penny's worth of niacin in their daily diet. It seems incredible that this deficiency took place in the world's wealthiest, most technologically advanced country during this century. If we were talking of a backward, third world country, it would be easier to accept. Niacin deficiency seems so trivial today that it's hard to grasp in retrospect how serious it was not very long ago. Niacin was given status as a B vitamin and named in 1948, and pellagra had been completely eliminated by 1945.

An interesting aside is worth mentioning. Niacin was deficient in the South because poor people relied almost completely on corn flour. The corn was processed without lime, as had been done for centuries in old Mexico. The presence of lime causes a minor chemical change in the corn flour that also releases niacin and makes it available for human absorption. So if mothers had used the old folkways of processing corn, the tragedy of pellagra never would have happened. Now the niacin and other nutrient problems are solved by fortification; that is, adding the nutrients back that were lost in processing.

THE B TEAM

Niacin, along with the six other B vitamins, is part of the B team. The game this team plays is metabolism. Metabolism controls all human energy, including that involved in the mental work of a crossword puzzle or the physical work of bridge building.

When one of these vitamins is missing, metabolism is disturbed. Poor metabolism shows up first in the most active tissue, the brain. But since mental decline can be so subtle and hard to recognize, the first physical symptom is the red skin of niacin deficiency. A redneck and someone displaying the behavior that follows, a "shade-tree sitter," are the same thing. Both terms emerged at the same time and persist today for mentally slow, lazy people. As a nutrient, niacin protects us from many serious physical illnesses, including mental decline.

NIACIN AND CHOLESTEROL

In 1989, *The 8-Week Cholesterol Cure* by Robert E. Kowalski swept the country. Everyone is concerned about cholesterol, and any book that promised an eight-week correction for a lifetime problem was bound to be a bestseller. This book introduced the average person to what scientists had known for a long time: Megadoses of niacin can lower cholesterol in most people.

Lowering cholesterol with niacin calls for taking 1 to 8 grams daily. That's 50 to 400 times the RDA of 20 milligrams daily. When niacin is used in such large amounts, it requires medical supervision. Niacin's side effects at the 3- to 8-gram level, though not life threatening, are difficult to tolerate. These side effects include nausea, severe flushing of the face, itching, and so forth. Nevertheless, niacin lowers cholesterol, is cheap compared to other drugs, and its side effects are not nearly as bad as those of other drugs, even though they're uncomfortable.

While cholesterol lowering might be the only quick-fix most people look for from niacin, it's emerging as one of nature's most important "fixers." For instance, working along with an important enzyme, niacin fixes broken genetic material. In this capacity niacin is a unique protector.

NIACIN THE PROTECTOR

Many things can cause a break in the genetic material of a cell, DNA. Cosmic rays left over from the origin of the universe or stars that exploded as supernovas millions of years ago cause DNA breaks. Common chemical DNA-breakers include oxides and some free radicals found in the air we breathe and the food we eat and the water we drink. Random breaks in DNA also show up when cells are dividing. Some number manipulation will help you see why DNA breaks are so important to life.

Breaks in DNA caused by cosmic rays occur very rarely. Take

a small number; let's say it happens only once in every ten million cell divisions; that's one in ten million. Stick with that small number and let only one break in ten million lead to a cancerous cell.

Now do some arithmetic. Say you have fifty trillion cells that divide, on average, once in seven weeks. Using the example of one in ten million times, gives you one hundred and eighty-five chances at cancer by age fifty, and the chances increase as we get older. That's a lot of opportunity to get cancer, so why don't we all get it? Because there's a system to correct these mistakes. Each cell that can divide has an elaborate system that corrects breaks in DNA.

A good analogy to this correction is the active beehive. If you cause a break in a beehive and can stick around to see what happens, you'd be amazed. Worker bees jump right in to repair the break. Some would make the waxy substance. Others would mold it into just the correct shape. In a short time the new compartments would be built. Then other bees fill them with honey and within a day or two you'd never know the hive was broken.

DNA breaks are similar, except they take place at a level even the most powerful electron microscope can't see. You can only watch the occurrence by elaborate biochemical techniques in very sophisticated laboratories. An enzyme system, named a DNA polymerase, steps in to repair the break. This enzyme uses niacin as its tool. In the beehive analogy, it's like the feet the worker bees use to shape the honeycomb. Niacin doesn't become part of the DNA, but without its activated form, the DNA wouldn't be repaired.

The same is true in the case of the beehive. Workers could make the wax, but without the other workers using their feet correctly, you'd only have beeswax and not an elaborate, well-shaped hive.

Myron (Mike) and Elaine Jacobson (a husband and wife team), respectively professors of biochemistry and medicine at the University of North Texas, are leaders in unraveling the marvelous biochemistry of DNA repair. There's no longer any debate about how it works or if it works; that's established. We're now focusing on how much niacin is needed to be sure it works effectively in humans. In their own words: "We don't know what the optimal levels of niacin are in the diet so people are protected against cancer. That's the current frontier."

The Jacobsons' findings about niacin haven't been converted to human epidemiology. But they have established the biochemistry so clearly, and the potential for mistakes in DNA is so obvious, that it's just a matter of time before epidemiologists bring it to a clear focus in terms of food. The findings underscore the fact that protection by some nutrients is not within their scope as vitamins. RDA levels of niacin could be sufficient for protection under most circumstances, but frankly, we don't know. With what we do know, anyone who doesn't pay attention to a good diet with enough niacin is foolish. Niacin is obtained readily in foods and food supplements.

GUARANTEEING DIETARY NIACIN

Brewers yeast is the best source of niacin in a comparison of foods based on weights. But don't rush out for a beer or a loaf of bread, because modern beer has had the yeast and solids that contain niacin removed and our bread is different than it was in the Middle Ages. A few simple food rules will, however, insure that you get enough niacin.

- Eat fish three times weekly. Eat white meat of poultry and occasionally lean red meat. They all provide 8 to 10 milligrams of niacin in a serving; that's 40 percent of the RDA.
- Follow the Longevity Diet in part four for cereals and whole grains. This gives you an additional 30 percent of niacin's RDA.
- Regularly eating beans gives you another 20 to 40 percent of niacin's RDA.
- Snack on nuts. An ounce of cashews, for example, has about 10 milligrams of niacin, or 50 percent of the RDA.
- If you use a supplement, be sure it contains niacin at 100 percent of the RDA.

12

Calcium and Sunshine

"Every child needs the January sun"
         —Folk wisdom, 13th-century Weistar, Germany

"A pinch of limestone to grow on"
         —Mexican folk wisdom about tortilla making, before A.D. 1000

The above two folk sayings reflect practices that helped insure the survival and healthy development of children for thousands of years. Each insured that children would build strong bones and teeth and not become crippled from poor bone growth at critical times. The first saying insured adequate vitamin D, and the second calcium.

Calcium and Sunshine Quiz

Answer yes or no to the following questions:

- Do you get fewer than three or four servings of dairy products every day?

- Do you have any blood relatives who seem to get shorter and hunched over as they age?

- Do you exercise fewer than five times weekly?

- Do you get less than thirty minutes of sunshine daily?

- Are you bothered by nagging low-back pain not traceable to muscle strain?

- Do you try to keep your cholesterol as low as possible?

A yes answer to any of these questions indicates you need to learn more about the importance of the mineral calcium and vitamin D, the sunshine vitamin.

MEETING CALCIUM NEEDS BEFORE THE MODERN ERA

Every successful society developed methods of getting enough calcium to suit its environment. Calcium is the only mineral required in large quantities. Milk and dairy products have always been among the best sources. However, there are other, equally good ways of getting calcium.

In old Mexico, over fifteen hundred years before European influence, corn was processed with utensils made of limestone, a calcium mineral. In addition, Mexican mothers added a pinch of limestone to each tortilla. Since the tortilla was an edible eating utensil made from corn, everyone got enough calcium. In other hot climates between the tropics of Cancer and Capricorn, fermented dairy products, such as yogurt and cheese, were the safest sources of calcium.

Nowadays we often wonder why the Mexicans and other societies didn't raise cows. Well, some of them simply didn't have grazing land for cows or, in some areas, the disease, tuberculosis, which is spread in milk, was a limiting factor. These people usually solved their calcium need in other ways, which were in harmony with their environment.

Vietnamese women dissolved bones from fish and chicken in a strong vinegar to make a sort of bone stock, much as some chefs do with chicken or beef stock today. This calcium-rich stock was added to just about every dish. So, as from the pinch of limestone in Mexico, everyone got enough calcium.

Sweet and sour cooking was yet another way to extract calcium from bones. The "sour," acidic part of the cooking leached calcium from the bones into the sauce. Consequently, what is now a pleasant, "ethnic" Chinese food in North America, actually began from more important health values.

CALCIUM TODAY: A MODERN SHORTFALL

Today, in North America, lack of calcium is a major, dietary problem. Our rich diet, with its abundance of protein and fat, coupled with our tall stature impose high calcium requirements: over 1,000 milligrams daily for an average adult.

About 1,000 milligrams of calcium per person enters our dietary system daily. That's just about enough to go around, but it usually doesn't go to the people who need it. Table 12.1 summarizes the calcium RDA for a few, key age groups and the amount of calcium government surveys indicate these people get from all dietary sources. Table 12.1 indicates that calcium shortfall is mostly a woman's problem.

TABLE 12.1

Calcium
Need and Dietary Reality

Actual Calcium Intake

Women's Age	Need	Need	Reality		Need
	RDA,* in milligrams per day	Medical** Recommendation	Actual Intake As: Percent of RDA	Percent of Medical Recommendation	Expressed As: Glasses of Milk
12 to 18	1200		69		4
19 to 34	1200		57		4
35 to 44	800	1000	75	60	2½ to 3
65 to 74	800	1500	68	36	2½ to 7
Men's Age					
65 to 74	800		87		2½

*Recommended Dietary Allowances, 10th Edition, 1989
**Medical Consensus Panel of the *Journal of the American Medical Association*

Table 12.1 teaches an important lesson: Women stop getting the RDA for calcium before age eighteen! In fact, by age fourteen, most girls fall below the RDA. Milk is usually dropped in favor of soft drinks or because girls think it's fattening.

In addition to setting the RDA, the government has called on panels of experts to recommend calcium levels for special groups. I've included two of their recommendations in table 12.1. Our shortfall in dietary calcium, when compared to these consensus recommendations, is serious. If you think of your bones as a calcium reservoir, these dietary shortfalls are disasters waiting to happen.

OSTEOPOROSIS: SIMPLE PROTECTION

Calcium does many jobs in your body. Calcium is so important that there's always about 10 milligrams in 100 milliliters of our blood. Calcium is essential for nerve function, blood pressure regulation, muscle contraction, acid-base balance, and many other things. In addition, calcium is necessary for the excretion of waste materials in the urine. Consequently, some is always lost in the urine. The water reservoir comparison is good for calcium. Some water in any reservoir is lost to evaporation, seepage into the soil, and leaks. So, even without any water use, the reservoir goes down a little each day if it's not replenished.

The calcium balance in your body is similar to the water in a water reservoir. On a daily basis, calcium loss is so small it's not noticed; just like a reservoir. At first, only the most sensitive instruments could detect the change. But after about twenty years of a little calcium loss from the bone reservoir, it becomes noticeable. It starts to show up in middle age in subtle ways; low-back pain, shorter stature, and hunched shoulders, to name a few. As the bones become less dense, they become weaker. When bones lose calcium, they're like wooden beams in a house that are slowly being eaten up by termites. On the outside you don't notice the change, but, after a while, a ceiling might cave in, a beam could crush in your hand, or a wall might cave in when you lean against it.

That's what happens with osteoporosis. Bones become more and more porous, like termite-eaten beams. The name is very descriptive; *osteo* means bones and *porosis* means porous. If the calcium shortfall most women experience between the ages of twelve and fifty isn't bad enough, the process accelerates at menopause, because hormone balance changes. This shift in hormone balance accelerates bone loss. Sticking with our reservoir analogy, it's as if the dam springs a leak and no one knows it; or, with the beams, it's as if another group of termites gets started.

At menopause, the body slows production of the hormone estrogen. Since estrogen is involved in building bones, it's as if the stream that fills the reservoir is diverted, and the loss accelerates. That's why osteoporosis was always thought of as a disease of aging. It usually makes its physical appearance a few years after menopause begins. Now we know it starts in the teenage years as a marginal nutrition deficiency. It just accelerates at menopause.

In osteoporosis, bones eventually become so weak they shatter like glass and are almost impossible to repair. We now believe that bones break and people fall; they don't fall and break their bones. Though not considered fatal, all the consequences of the broken bones are often so devastating that many elderly women never recover fully and often some die. Broken bones from osteoporosis are a leading cause of death in elderly women.

Even if the doctor prescribes estrogen supplements at menopause to stop the bone loss, you still need calcium. In fact, many medical scientists agree that you need 1,500 milligrams of calcium daily, the same as you'd get from five glasses of milk, along with estrogen; without estrogen, 2,000 milligrams of calcium daily (that's almost seven glasses of milk). This is where the consensus panel recommendation came from in table 12.1. However, calcium won't always be effective without estrogen. The only way to be sure is for your doctor to make several bone density measurements over about twelve months. If the bone density decline continues in spite of enough calcium, take action by using estrogen.

Once menopause begins, the use of estrogen and other drugs is a medical issue. However, you always need calcium. It is always a dietary and preventive need before and after menopause. You never outgrow your need for calcium, even if you outgrow your desire to drink milk. If bones aren't enough reason for calcium, the other sections of this chapter should convince you.

Some women avoid taking estrogen because they fear it will increase the likelihood of their getting cancer. Though it does increase the risk slightly, doctors can determine who is at greatest risk and take measures to reduce that risk. Modern medicine can do much to stop bone loss and improve bone density, but it always requires calcium.

OSTEOPOROSIS CAN BE PREVENTED

Osteoporosis is not a disease of aging! Osteoporosis is a marginal nutritional deficiency disease that starts in youth and whose effects show up around age fifty. It can be prevented at any time along the way. Prevention is your responsibility. It begins with getting sufficient dietary calcium, all the other nutrients, and exercise. Yes, exercise!

If you don't use it, you lose it! If you force your bones to work and you eat right, your body rises to the need and builds strong bones. If you don't require much from your body, it won't give much. In short, weight-bearing exercise causes your body to build strong bones. So exercise is important and you never outgrow the need for it.

Astronauts make a good case for exercise. As soon as they enter the weightlessness of space, their bones start releasing calcium. After all, it takes energy and nutrients from the body to maintain strong bones. You don't need strong bones in space, so the primitive part of our brain says: "You're not using it, so I'll let it go." That's why every prolonged stay in space, by anyone, includes exercise. It's not just to prove astronauts stay in shape for a segment on the evening news.

Besides exercise, you can avoid foods or habits that increase calcium loss. These include taking in excess caffeine, meat, alcohol, and smoking.

Oriental diets are more nearly vegetarian than ours. Though Oriental people are usually of shorter stature, they get along and thrive on proportionately less calcium than people in North America. Our increased need for calcium seems to result from the excess phosphorus in our diet. Most of it comes from the abundance of meat and poultry that we eat. Soft drinks are another source of phosphorus. That's why they were originally called "phosphates."

Dr. Tony Albanese, now an octogenarian, and a leader in bone-restorative studies using calcium supplements, studied the effect of the calcium-to-phosphorus ratio on bone density. Dr. Albanese found that a diet with a calcium-to-phosphorus ratio of one is probably best; and the closer to one or more, the better. You don't have to become chemists. You only need to follow some easy rules.

STEPS TO PREVENT OSTEOPOROSIS

• *Follow the Longevity Diet!* It has the right calcium to phosphorus ratio.

• *Calcium:* Strive for 1,000 milligrams daily before menopause; 1,500 milligrams daily after menopause. A thousand milligrams of calcium requires drinking three and a half 8-ounce glasses of milk or eating three 6-ounce servings of yogurt; 1,500 milligrams calls for a 50-percent increase in these amounts. See table 12.2, at the end of this chapter, for the best sources of calcium.

• *Calcium supplements:* If you rely on supplements for your calcium, use equal amounts made from calcium carbonate or limestone and calcium phosphate. You should also select calcium supplements that contain magnesium. Calcium supplements should be taken at mealtimes with food, especially carbohydrates.

• *Foods in moderation:* Coffee, soft drinks, alcohol, and meat, especially red and organ meats.

• *Exercise:* Do weight-bearing exercise daily; climb stairs, take out garbage, bring in the shopping. Don't count jumping to conclusions, but jumping rope is excellent.

THE OSTEOPOROSIS EPIDEMIC

A great deal has been written about osteoporosis, so I've given you only the salient features. However, you should recognize that there's a major osteoporosis epidemic among postmenopausal women and it's appearing in men as well. The cure for osteoporosis is an excellent example of how prevention works and proof that you're never too old to make a difference.

One of Dr. Albanese's best studies was conducted on women whose average age was eighty-two. He proved that with exercise and calcium, they could improve their bone density. His research proves how resilient our bodies are and that we are never too old to improve our health. In this particular study, he took away even the excuse of ''I'm too old.''

DOES CALCIUM DO MORE?

Sufficient calcium is required to maintain nervous system function, normal blood pressure, and muscle strength. It's not by accident that the body works hard to maintain a constant level of calcium in the blood, even if it has to do it at the expense of our bones. Calcium's effect on blood is important.

Some people are so sensitive to the level of calcium in their blood that if it drops below the RDA, their blood pressure slowly increases by 10 to 15 percent. A 10-percent rise in blood pressure causes many people with "normal" blood pressure to have high blood pressure or hypertension and increases the likelihood of an early death. Fortunately for these people, two extra glasses of milk daily will usually reverse the increase in blood pressure. In clinical studies, doctors use calcium supplements, but milk, yogurt, or cheese also works. Some evidence suggests these people need more calcium than the RDA of 800 or 1,000 milligrams. So if you've got mild hypertension, why not stretch your calcium intake to 1,200 milligrams daily. Now let's explore how calcium helps prevent colon cancer.

When I tell people we only absorb about 35 percent of the calcium in our diet, they're astounded. I quickly add that the Creator doesn't waste things; she puts the other 65 percent to work. This excess intestinal calcium helps regulate many things, but, most of all, it reduces our chances of getting colorectal cancer. People listen, because I've never met anyone who wants to get cancer.

At least one bile acid has been identified, in 1940, as a weak carcinogen. That is, it causes cancer. It's an irritant, just like the materials in betel nuts and smoking that cause cells to become dysplastic, then cancerous.

Dietary fat promotes cancer. That's why experts always say you should reduce fat. Although dietary fiber helps to neutralize the effects of both dietary fat and bile acids in promoting cancer, calcium also helps. Calcium has a simple but effective role in this neutralization of fats and bile acids. It combines with them to form insoluble "soaps."

A soap, as defined by a chemist, forms when calcium links up with a large fatty acid, like the kind you get from beef, pork, homogenized milk, or cheese. Calcium soaps are also formed with the bile acids. These calcium soaps don't dissolve in water. When you get adequate dietary fiber, they are swept out in the stools. All this adds up to a simple truth: get enough calcium and fiber to help eliminate excess fat and bile acids.

Calcium also imparts a modest cholesterol-lowering effect because of its action on fat. I learned about this in 1978 when Dr. Tony Albanese was doing a study to improve bone density with calcium supplements. While looking at the blood chemistry results, I noticed that the cholesterol level in women on calcium dropped, in comparison with that of the women on the placebo, whose cholesterol remained the same. I asked Tony if he was aware of this, and he said the cholesterol always drops in these studies because the calcium soaps remove bile acids and fat. Removing bile acids and fat is indirectly the same as removing cholesterol from your blood. So there's an added bonus with calcium.

CANCER

When epidemiologists observed that dietary calcium reduced the risk of intestinal cancer, their first thought was that the calcium forms calcium soaps and prevents the irritation-dysplastic cancer sequence. To many scientists, it was the end of the story. Then several scientists looked at vitamin D just to be sure. Lo and behold, they saw that vitamin D was also involved in reducing cancer risk. Calcium and vitamin D together prevent cancer.

People who live in sunbelt states have slightly lower rates of intestinal cancer than those who live in northern states. When this finding turned up, scientists first thought the difference must be vitamin D. Research has since shown that marginal amounts of vitamin D in the blood predispose us toward intestinal cancer. Add this to the findings about calcium and a team emerges. I call this team "partners in prevention." But let's take a diversion into the romance of the sunshine vitamin.

THE SUNSHINE VITAMIN

Since the streets were narrow and the windows in their homes were so small, women in thirteenth-century Weistar, Germany, would take their infants outdoors and expose them nude to the sun for a short time every day. They knew this was essential for good health.

After all, their mothers had said, "Every child needs the January sun."

Anthropological analysis of bones from the cemetery and church records show that a child who wasn't exposed to the sun either became deformed or died. So if a child was born in the fall and was still frail in January, or was sick and couldn't be exposed to the sun, that child had a lower chance of survival or of a normal life.

When ultraviolet rays in sunshine fall on your skin, they convert cholesterol in your blood to vitamin D. Vitamin D is essential for the body to absorb calcium from food. Therefore the infant who got no sun actually suffered from serious calcium deficiency. Breast milk has no vitamin D, so nursing the infant wouldn't help. Since the body only makes the vitamin D it needs and the excess is toxic, our bodies evolved so we relied on sunshine, and not mother's milk, to get enough.

Vitamin-D deficiency causes calcium deficiency even though it's really sunlight deficiency. The disease is called rickets in children and osteomalacia in adults. You can suffer and even die from vitamin D deficiency at any age, but growing children and pregnant and nursing women are most vulnerable.

In some societies pregnant and nursing women were restricted from public view and usually remained indoors. This taboo led to a folk saying: "Every child costs a tooth." This saying was based on a dental problem that developed in these women because the aveolar bone of their lower jaw, in which the teeth were fastened, gave up calcium easily. The mother's teeth would loosen, periodontal infection would follow, and good-bye tooth. Wealthy people with a secluded courtyard didn't have the tooth-loss problem because a pregnant or nursing woman could get the sun without being seen in public.

Nowadays we fortify milk, because a problem emerged during our industrial revolution similar to one that arose in England during their industrial revolution. Factory smoke would blot out the sun, and children who spent much time indoors during school or in factory work wouldn't get enough sunlight. Consequently, in 1921, over 21 percent of the children in American cities had signs of rickets. Fortifying milk with vitamin D solved this problem. It eliminated rickets by 1926. Other countries do the same thing, and whenever they've stopped fortification, rickets reappears.

Vitamin D is essential to transport calcium from the intestines into the blood. In the process, it enters the cells that line the intestines. So, no vitamin D is to calcium what ocean water is to the sailor at sea. To quote from Coleridge's *Rime of the Ancient Mariner:* "Water, water everywhere / Nor any drop to drink."

CALCIUM AND VITAMIN D

We know that vitamin D activates calcium in the cells that line the intestines. In addition, studies on high blood pressure, studies on nerve cell function, and on muscle contraction teach us that calcium has an important regulatory role at the cellular level. Could calcium's role for preventing cancer go beyond its ability to form soaps? Yes, otherwise vitamin D wouldn't be involved with calcium.

It's the same old story. Calcium must get inside some cells. For this to happen, vitamin D is essential. Once inside, calcium helps regulate things so the cells don't become dysplastic. If they already have, the presence of calcium makes them revert to normal. Are we seeing the folic acid story played out again? I think it comes close.

CALCIUM THE REGULATOR

But this story is a little different from the folic acid story. Calcium has a two-faced role in our intestines. Its first face forms calcium soaps, neutralizes irritants like bile acids, and removes cancer promoters, such as saturated fatty acids. Its second face is more complex. It works inside each individual cell to keep it healthy and regulate its growth.

High blood pressure and cancer risk emerge when calcium's regulatory role can't be realized because of calcium deficiency from a poor diet. Both effects call for enough calcium and vitamin D so calcium can enter each cell in sufficient quantity to work. It's that simple.

THE COLOR OF VITAMIN D

Excessive vitamin D is toxic to the point of death. Therefore, you'd expect our body to have a regulatory system to protect us. It does. It makes a pigment, melanin, for the job.

People who developed in equatorial regions have thick, black skin. The rich pigment and skin thickness prevent too much ultraviolet light from penetrating to the blood, so too much vitamin D isn't made. This pigment also protects these people from skin cancer.

People living further north can develop a dark tan when the sun gets high in the sky during the summer, but become light again during the long winter months when the sun is low in the sky. The skin of these people isn't quite as thick as that of those from the equatorial regions.

People living in the far north, for example, Scotland or Lapland, have light, thin skin. This allows their body to get enough U.V. rays from the low, summer sun and store enough vitamin D for the long winter. Some of these people tan very slowly, and some, such as Scots, don't tan at all.

Besides getting sunlight, another approach was using fish oils, a method that had the dual advantage of providing both vitamins A and D. So not surprisingly, the ritual of eating fish once weekly went from a folk custom for personal survival in northern climates to a religious practice for group survival. Indeed, it became sinful if not practiced. It even showed up in childrens' songs that went like this: "Friday fish for all you hungry men." The dietary need for calcium and vitamin D led to sun worship, folk wisdom, and serious religious practice.

GETTING ENOUGH CALCIUM

You've read that excessive sunlight causes skin cancer. Let's put our need for vitamin D and sunshine in perspective. Thirty minutes of partial exposure—say, the face, arms, and shoulders—to sunlight each day is not excessive. If you get that much you won't need to fear skin cancer, and you'll get more than enough vitamin D.

Milk, dairy products, and many calcium supplements are fortified with vitamin D. So with a little prudent planning, you will always have enough vitamin D.

Dairy products are the most readily available sources of calcium. However, dairy products often mean plenty of calories and fat, so I've listed the amount of calcium in various dairy products and the number of calories required to get 100 milligrams of calcium; then I've listed some vegetable sources of calcium along with them. Always remember, you can't eat too many vegetables.

TABLE 12.2

Calcium Sources

Source	Amount	Calcium, in milligrams	Calories per 100 milligrams of calcium
Milk			
Skim milk	8 ounces	302	30
2% Milk	8 ounces	297	40
Whole milk	8 ounces	316	50
Yogurt			
Yogurt, low fat	8 ounces	452	28
Yogurt, whole	8 ounces	274	51
Cheese			
Cheddar cheese	1 ounce	204	56
Cottage cheese, creamed	4 ounces	68	172
Cottage cheese, low fat	8 ounces	138	118
Feta cheese	1 ounce	140	54
Mozzarella cheese	1 ounce	147	54
Ricotta cheese, low fat	4 ounces	337	51
Brie cheese	1 ounce	52	182
Vegetables			
Beans, boiled	1 cup	100	241
Kale	½ cup	90	22
Cabbage	½ cup	16	50
Broccoli	½ cup	21	57
Blackeyed peas	1 cup	42	471
Seaweed	3.5 ounces	168	26
Spinach	½ cup	28	21

Meat and Fish			
Red meat, lean	3.5 ounces	7	3,000
Clams/oysters, steamed	3.5 ounces	78	161
Bread			
Whole-wheat bread	1 slice	23	291

A quick review of table 12.2 indicates that dairy products are the best sources of calcium. Low-fat dairy products supply as much calcium as high-fat and have fewer calories. With the exception of creamed cottage cheese, cheese and yogurt are excellent sources of calcium.

Vegetables such as broccoli, cabbage, and spinach, are excellent sources of calcium. Simply take extra helpings of these and other deep-green vegetables. There aren't enough calories to concern you and the protective value is outstanding.

CALCIUM SUPPLEMENTS

If you don't get about 800 milligrams of calcium from dairy products and don't studiously strive to get it from other sources, you should use calcium supplements. Now, how to select the right supplement.

• Choose a supplement that supplies 150 to 350 milligrams of calcium per tablet. It should also contain magnesium, another mineral, which is usually insufficient in supply if your calcium level is low.

• Don't take more than about 400 milligrams of calcium as a supplement at a meal. If you take too much at one time, you won't absorb 35 percent. You'll probably absorb only about 15 percent. Absorption of any nutrient is less efficient when there's too much.

• Take calcium supplements at mealtime because food, especially carbohydrates, helps with calcium absorption.

CALCIUM FROM FOOD

Getting enough calcium from food isn't difficult, but it requires care:

• *Milk:* Use 8 ounces of low-fat milk on cereal every day.

- *Dairy products:* Select low-fat yogurt or cheese regularly.

- *Vegetables:* Select dark green ones. Take an extra serving, as the calories are insignificant and the nutritional value outstanding.

- *Snacks:* Use hard cheese sparingly. One ounce of hard cheese goes a long way.

- *Fortified foods:* Calcium-fortified foods, such as orange juice, are practical.

PART

III

PROTECTOR FOODS

In 1989, when President George Bush declared that he didn't like broccoli, he dealt preventive health a low blow. Broccoli, one of the cruciferous vegetables, helps prevent cancer and is a good source of vitamin C and fiber. When a national leader declares that he doesn't like a food like broccoli, he gives lots of people, especially children, an excuse not to eat it.

In this short section, you'll encounter two food groups, garlic and the cruciferous vegetables, which provide a powerful, preventive impact. By making a habit of eating foods from each group regularly and abundantly, you can do a lot for your own health and the health of those you care about.

Food and lifestyle habits form the basis of longevity. Some scientists claim we understand nutrition so well that we can put everything a person needs into a "food bag" and keep them free from any nutritional deficiencies. This position implicitly accepts the classical nutrition-deficiency symptoms as the criteria for need: if you don't show deficiency symptoms, you're getting enough of the nutrient. This book is based on another criteria: the quality and quantity of life can be enhanced by prevention of major and minor diseases.

Cruciferous vegetables, garlic, onions, shallots, and leeks are examples of vegetables that help prevent cancer, high blood pressure, stroke, and even modulate blood sugar levels. In addition, we know that if they help prevent cancer and high blood pressure, they shore up our defenses against myriad illnesses that are not catastrophic when compared to cancer. However, these comparatively minor illnesses, such as emphysema, asthma, and minor infections, detract from the quality of life. And there is evidence suggesting they have a cumulative life-shortening effect, albeit minor.

So, as you read the next two chapters, keep in mind that our criteria for health are relative to a point in history. When plagues were the most feared killers, the simple antibiotic properties of garlic were magical. Later, when fear shifted to the niacin-deficiency disease pellagra (chapter 11), the curative powers of rice hulls or beans seemed magical until we identified a few vitamins. The fear of those diseases has been replaced by the fear of cancer. In the fight against cancer, as proved true in the battles against the plague, scurvy, pellagra, and others, prevention is king. In that context, these vegetables have a few properties that seem magical today but before too long will be reduced to some identifiable chemicals and components. Even after that identification, it will still be best to eat the vegetables. Food will always be the vehicle of prevention, and prevention will always rule.

13

Garlic, Onions, Leeks, and Shallots Too

"And, most dear actors, eat no onions or garlick; for we are to utter sweet breath . . ."
—Shakespeare, *A Midsummer Night's Dream*

Garlic is a perennial herb and a member of the lily family. Its relatives include onions, chives, leeks, autumn crocus, and lily of the valley, among many others. Garlic, native to Central Asia, where it grows wild, was cultivated all over the world before 3000 B.C. This makes it one of the oldest cultivated plants, and it is impossible to identify its beginnings.

Garlic has been indispensable in Chinese cooking for over four thousand years. In Egypt, laborers who built the pyramids of Cheops in 2800 B.C. were given a daily clove of garlic for strength. Six garlic bulbs were found in Tutankhamen's tomb, which dates from 1300 B.C. The garlic was placed there by his priests either to ward off evil spirits or for him to use on his otherworldly journey. By that time, the Egyptians had recognized garlic's medicinal value.

Codex Ebers, an Egyptian medical papyrus written in 1550 B.C., gives over eight hundred therapeutic formulas. Twenty-two of them use garlic and others include garlic. Over one thousand years later, in 450 B.C., Hippocrates ranked garlic as one of the most important of his "four hundred simples" or therapeutic remedies.

217

> ### Garlic, Onion, Leek, and
> ### Shallot Quiz

Answer yes or no to the following questions:

- Do you add fresh garlic, onions, shallots, or chives to foods and salads?

- Have you or a blood relative had high blood pressure or blood sugar troubles?

- Do you believe that fresh garlic will keep vampires from attacking?

- Do you believe that garlic and onions can help prevent colds and fight infections?

Whether you answer yes or no to any of these questions, I think you'll find this chapter interesting and helpful.

Garlic is an English name derived from Old English words that mean "leek spear." Garlic's botanic name, *Allium sativum,* means "pungent wild herb." Garlic has its own name in most languages, verifying its age and diversity. For example, French *ail,* German *knoblauch,* Spanish *ajo,* and Italian *aglio.* But its Greek folk name, *thēriakē,* poor-man's treacle, hints at its broad value even to this day.

Poor-man's treacle is the most widely used name for garlic. Treacle is simply translated from Greek to "antidote," the use that transcends national boundaries and is global. For example, when Stalin asked musicians to write music for the state, "treacle" was actually worked into a song depicting the needs of peasants. Most "therapeutic" effects are now understood in the light of modern science, but for the peasants, garlic was truly wondrous. So, "antidote" was a pretty good name for them to give garlic. More importantly, garlic is still a protective food for the twenty-first century.

GARLIC IN FOLKLORE

Twentieth-century scientists have identified some of garlic's active chemical components. What's most revealing from this research is that it confirms the accuracy of folklore and proves that many old wives' tales are correct.

Since research has been so supportive of garlic's rich folklore, I chose to discuss folk use in the light of modern science. I hope you'll gain new respect for garlic, have a healthy desire to eat more of it in your food, and develop a high regard for folk wisdom.

I have but one reservation for you. In our ancestors' time, garlic's properties bordered on the magical and they used garlic for therapeutic purposes. Nowadays we have drugs, but it's important to see these properties of garlic as protective and as a reason to use it regularly in food. These protective properties will produce a longer, healthier life.

FOUR THIEVES VINEGAR, 1721

Four condemned criminals were "volunteered" to bury dead bodies during the great bubonic plague of Marseilles in 1721. It was actually an unspoken death sentence, because they were expected to get the plague. Much to the surprise of court officials, the convict gravediggers never got the plague. Their immunity resulted from the use of a folk remedy, which consisted of wine laced with crushed garlic. In their honor, this concoction has since been known as "Four Thieves Vinegar," even though the concoction was known long before 1721. It is actually made by adding garlic to wine, although it would also work with vinegar. Garlic's ability to kill bacteria—although not stated as such—was identified in the Codex Ebers of 1550 B.C., in which it was listed as being used to clean wounds, especially from animal bites.

In 1858, Louis Pasteur, who identified bacteria as the agents of infection, proved that garlic juice is antibacterial—that is, it would kill bacteria. In 1913, Albert Schweitzer used garlic juice for sterilizing wounds in his hospital at Lambarene, Africa. During both wars, but mostly in World War I, garlic juice was used to clean, sterilize, and dress wounds. During World War I, the English government paid one shilling per pound for garlic to supply field hospitals. In those days, one shilling was beyond all reason for a pound of vegetables, but not for a drug. The price confirms that garlic was used as a medication and not as a food.

In 1944, Chester J. Cavallito published the results of his research proving that garlic juice is an effective antibiotic against a number of pathogenic microorganisms. In 1944, World War II was in full swing and the need for antibiotics was intense. Penicillin, discovered only four years previously, was being produced for the war efforts and there was an intensive search for other natural antibiotics. Fungi from which commercial antibiotics are produced can be grown in large vats and harvested in large quantities year round in any location. So garlic didn't become a commercial source of antibiotics, because it must be grown as a crop. But garlic was practical for common folks, while the fungal antibiotics are not.

Garlic juice diluted to one part in 125,000 prevents the growth of the following pathogenic bacteria: staphylococcus, streptococcus, vibrio (cholera), bacillus (typhus), bacillus dysenteriae (dysenteria), bacillus enteritis (enteric infections). For bacillus typhus, diluted garlic juice is better than penicillin!

One part in 125,000 is the equivalent of about one teaspoonful of garlic juice in 162 gallons! In short, when you can easily extract enough garlic juice to fill a teaspoon, you've got a material that prevents the growth of many deadly germs.

The juice is also effective against many pathogenic fungi and yeasts; for example, the yeasts that cause common vaginitis. In recent years, scientists have found that garlic juice is also effective against influenza B and herpes-simplex type-I viruses.

In 1990, the first international conference on the therapeutic effects of garlic was held in Washington, D.C. At the conference, a Chinese scientist explained how garlic oil is injected directly into the blood of people with resistant fungus infections. Though this practice seems primitive in view of the excellent antifungal agents available today, it is probably the limit of how far effective folk remedies can be carried.

Cavallito proved that garlic's active antibacterial ingredients come from sulfur-containing materials that dissolve in alcohol and water and are partially responsible for its odor. Allicin, the most common, is volatile: that means it evaporates into the air. We'll see later that other materials in onions and garlic are both volatile and irritating to the eyes. It's the volatility of these active materials that makes another folk practice effective.

In cold weather, mothers often strung garlic cloves around children's necks to prevent the flu. Most flu and colds are caused by influenza B viruses that enter the body through the nose and mouth. Since the volatile materials in garlic kills these viruses, it follows that this practice must have been fairly effective. If everyone did it, garlic odor wouldn't be a problem, because everyone would smell the same.

With this excellent hindsight, you won't be surprised to learn that the following folk practices, some of which date to 1550 B.C., were also effective:

- Garlic poultice for infections

- Garlic lotion for pimples and boils

- Garlic in the stocking or shoe for whooping cough

- Crushed garlic on the soles of the feet, which are then wrapped in linen, to alleviate measles

You can do a simple experiment to prove how some of these remedies work. Have someone rub a garlic clove on the soles of your feet. In a few minutes you will taste garlic. Through the process of percutaneous absorption—absorption through the skin—the active ingredients in garlic enter the blood and go to all parts of the body. Wrapping your feet after covering them with crushed garlic for a day or so exceeded the level of allicin required to kill enough of the infectious organisms so that normal body defenses could take over and defeat the illness.

Garlic poultices could have sterilized a wound or killed the infection that caused a boil. Indeed, even if the boil had not opened, the active ingredients in garlic could penetrate the skin.

Garlic doesn't work on all infectious agents, as deaths from the great plagues proved. Research has proven that garlic juice will kill only some pathogenic organisms. An old childhood rhyme, "Ring Around the Rosy," verifies garlic's limits, since it describes burst boils (ring around the rosy), the use of flowers to cover the stench (a pocketful of posies), the cosmetic cover-up with ashes, and the last line (we all fall dead) describes the outcome. Isn't it amazing how accurate folklore is and how this childhood song reflects bygone reality? In France, many deaths were prevented by mixing garlic with wine and cleaning wounds with garlic. In fact, the French priests survived the great plague by using "Four Thieves Vinegar," but the English did not use it as the song indicates.

GARLIC CURES HOT BLOOD

High blood pressure is a widespread, modern, dietary disease related to excessive dietary salt, overweight, and inactivity. About 23 percent of North Americans have high blood pressure. Long before processed food, 2 to 5 percent of the people in any society developed high blood pressure. People who develop high blood pressure have minor but perceptible symptoms. Headaches and nosebleeds are the most common symptoms, but high blood pressure leads to heart disease, kidney failure, and visual problems. So even though blood pressure wasn't routinely measured by doctors until this century, people had symptoms when it became too high. In folk wisdom, these symptoms for high blood pressure were usually called "hot blood."

People knew that hot blood was bad. Folk remedies to cure hot blood included garlic. Though I've never had the opportunity to explore the numerous other plant remedies that are found in most countries and islands, it would be a good bet that many of the plants belong to the garlic and onion family.

Many modern drugs lower high blood pressure. Lowering high blood pressure is one of the largest pharmaceutical industries today. In the United States alone, it accounts for more than $10 billion annually. However, to Hippocrates in 450 B.C., garlic was one of the few agents that was effective.

In 1921, Dr. Michael Leoper published a paper discussing the blood-pressure-lowering effects of a garlic extract. It not only lowered blood pressure, but it relieved symptoms, such as headaches, dizziness, and occasional nosebleeds.

Other researchers at the time credited the effects of garlic on intestinal putrefaction. If indeed toxins from intestinal microbes have any role in high blood pressure, garlic could be effective because of its antibacterial properties or because it reduced the absorption of the toxins. The possibility that intestinal microbes can cause high blood pressure is still being researched.

In these studies, the clinicians used dehydrated garlic equivalent to 18 grams of fresh garlic or about ⅔ ounce and divided it into three daily doses. In more everyday terms, that's about one medium garlic clove taken three times a day.

Garlic also lowers blood pressure because some of its components cause the blood vessel walls to relax and dilate, reducing resistance to blood flow. We call this effect "reducing peripheral resistance." These same components also cause the kidney to reduce its output of high-blood-pressure-causing hormones. So it works a second way.

If all that isn't enough, garlic is a diuretic. A diuretic causes the kidneys to relax their reabsorption of salt and produce more urine. As they produce more urine, they release more salt, and this reduces blood pressure. Potassium, a second and necessary mineral, is also released, but since garlic supplies potassium, it naturally compensates, to some extent, for the loss. In 1985, Dr. Ed Block identified a material in garlic named ajoene that is responsible for lowering blood pressure. He then confirmed his findings by making the same material in the lab and testing it on people with high blood pressure. His findings have been expanded since then.

In this last decade of the twentieth century, high blood pressure is well understood. Over 80 percent of high blood pressure can be controlled by diet alone. Garlic can make the diet more effective and should be part of any dietary program. Its only side effect is a slightly pungent breath. Compared to most modern medications that produce dizzy spells, blackouts, and loss of sexual ability, to name three, a little garlic breath doesn't seem so bad.

GARLIC: HEART ATTACK AND APOPLEXY

Folklore is very clear on the use of garlic to prevent heart attack and stroke. In 3000 B.C., the Indian healer Charaka said garlic maintains the ability of blood to flow and strengthens the heart. Charaka is the father of Ayurvedic medicine, which is becoming widely practiced in North America, and teaches natural healing.

Hippocrates used garlic in 450 B.C. for people who either had had a heart attack or whom he felt were likely to have one. By the start of the Christian era, garlic was widely used for people with bad hearts. Now we know why garlic is so effective at preventing heart attacks and how it works.

If you form a blood clot inside a blood vessel and it blocks a vessel in your heart, you have a heart attack. If the clot blocks a vessel in your head, you have a stroke. The event itself is caused by the blood supply not getting to that part of the heart or brain served by the blocked vessel. A large clot can cut off a large enough vessel so the heart attack or stroke is massive enough to cause death. In fact, about 36 percent of all deaths are from a heart attack or stroke.

An internal blood clot is similar to the little scab that forms when you prick or scratch your skin, the only difference being that it has formed somewhere inside your body. It's theorized that the internal clot develops as a result of some physical or emotional stress. Physical trauma, such as a bruise, can injure a vessel to get the clot started. Physical and emotional stress cause our adrenal glands to produce the hormone adrenaline, which induces the body to form clots more easily. This is part of the body's defense system and stress raises all our defenses. So clot formation is a natural phenomenon involving natural materials produced in our body itself.

Actual clot development is a complex process starting with specialized blood cells called platelets. Along with platelets, an elaborate enzyme system and several proteins, especially a protein named fibrin, are required.

Platelets clump together to get the clot started. Then the protein fibrin becomes involved to build the clot matrix. Fibrin development is the clot development. Platelet aggregation is an indication of your risk of having a stroke. More aggregation is equated to greater risk.

We know today that stroke or heart attack risk increases with a reduced clotting time, beginning with high platelet aggregation. Risk of stroke and heart attack increase in proportion to higher blood pressure because high blood pressure forces platelets to clump more easily. Smoking, high blood fat, and high blood sugar all increase the risk of stroke and heart attack, because they increase platelet aggregation. That's why risk is highest right after a heavy, high-fat meal. Two or three of these risk factors together aren't just added together; they're multiplied by each other, so you should try to keep them all low.

Clinical studies prove that folklore about garlic was correct. Garlic contains materials that reduce both platelet clumping and fibrin activity. Therefore, it works by reducing both types of risk that cause internal clots to form. Add to that its ability to reduce blood pressure, and garlic becomes a one-plant task force against heart attack and stroke.

Several lines of evidence had supported this conclusion. Many people, especially some Indian vegetarians, eat lots of garlic, two or three ounces each week. Some consume moderate amounts of an ounce of garlic and others eat absolutely none. So, Dr. Gupta Sainani and his group of researchers at the Poona Medical College in India did the logical epidemiological analysis. They studied platelet clumping and fibrin activity in people and compared them to their garlic-eating habits. Both platelet clumping and fibrin activity decreased in proportion to increased garlic consumption. High-volume garlic consumers had the lowest rate of platelet aggregation and clot formation, while non-garlic consumers had the highest rate of platelet aggregation. The moderate garlic consumers had intermediate clotting tendencies.

Sainani's epidemiological studies have been confirmed in clinics where volunteers would consume garlic for a certain period of time; then they would consume no garlic, with an appropriate control period of a bland diet to allow the body to adjust. Both platelet clumping and fibrin activity rates decreased during high garlic consumption and increased when the garlic was removed.

Although garlic is one of the few plants that contain appreciable amounts of omega-3 oils, these oils don't account for the effects above. Even though the omega-3 oil, EPA, helps to reduce platelet clumping, it has no effect on fibrin activity.

You might become alarmed and ask, ''Could I eat so much garlic that my clotting tendency declines altogether?'' The answer is a firm no! Natural foods like garlic or fish oil can help reduce this clotting tendency only to an optimum level. After that they seem to have no further effect. It's as if there's a built-in safety factor so that you can't exceed safe levels with natural foods like garlic; sort of a grand design. You'd have to simply eat raw garlic all the time to be at risk, and you simply can't do it!

Another way to see this is to reconsider the Greenlanders. Their diet consists almost exclusively of sea mammals. You'd think that they would get so much EPA their blood wouldn't clot at all. Obviously, that's not the way it works, because they're perfectly normal and when they cut a finger, a scab forms just as it does for us.

Our North American diet predisposes us to be at higher risk for stroke and heart attack because our tendency for internal clot formation is higher. That's why doctors often tell men over forty-five to take an aspirin a day. Aspirin reduces the tendency of blood to clot internally in people who are at high risk. Eating lots of garlic and onions simply reduces this tendency toward stroke and heart attack naturally. An aspirin a day works, but it's not the natural way.

It's important to also consider that there are only two side effects from the use of garlic: bad breath and an occasional headache if you eat too much. The headache is a built-in limiting factor so you'll never get too much. In contrast, consider aspirin, the simplest drug, which is routinely given for a variety of reasons. A single aspirin causes your digestive system to lose about a third of a teaspoon of blood. In contrast, garlic helps protect your digestive system from cancer.

"GARLIC STOPS CANCER TUMORS"

In 1550 B.C., Codex Ebers reported that garlic stopped the growth of tumors. Its use against tumors persisted through the Asian, Greek, and Roman civilizations; the Romans also passed it to the English. Both English and Chinese folklore teaches that garlic keeps the stomach and intestines healthy, exactly where it seems to protect most.

In 1983, a paper entitled "Onion and Garlic Oils Inhibit Tumor Promotion" appeared in an English journal. This was the first step in using modern science to prove that Codex Ebers is correct. Other scientists devoted to eradicating cancer began two lines of research. In Houston, Dr. Michael Wargovich began studying the effects of garlic on tumors in animals. At the same time, a medical group in China began to search for a relationship between garlic consumption and cancer. Both avenues of research have come together with an inescapable conclusion: Folklore is correct. The active materials in garlic have anticancer properties. Put another way, these active materials are part of a growing class of chemicals we call chemo-preventive chemicals, chemicals that prevent cancer.

Biochemists focus on cancers that are well understood and can be studied with precision in experimental animals. What has emerged from this research suggests that allicin and some of its analogous materials protect the cell from damage by a number of cancer-causing agents. These cancer-causing agents include nitrosamines, hydrocarbons, and gamma irradiation from cobalt-60. To give you an idea of how dangerous these materials are, 100 percent of the experimental animals that are given the carcinogen or irradiation get cancer.

Either garlic oil, the active ingredient allicin, or materials analogous to allicin derived from garlic reduced cancer in proportion to their dose. At high doses, garlic is 100 percent effective! In other words, it reduced the cancer to zero in these experiments. This research proves that garlic oils are preventive and need to be taken before exposure to a cancer-causing agent for maximum benefit. It's most obvious in the case of radiation, where giving the garlic after exposure is not effective at all.

One word says it all: Prevention!

Skeptics always ask, "Okay, I won't let my rats eat nitrosamines or stand in front of gamma-ray emitters. Will eating garlic help me?" The epidemiologists say clearly: "Yes, it will!"

In Shadong, China, stomach cancer occurs at a high rate, but not everyone gets it. So epidemiologists studied dietary relationships to see if there was any food in the diet that reduced the rate of stomach cancer in people who seemed to be safe. What they searched for was the consumption of a single food that would show an inverse relationship to cancer. In other words, the more you ate of the food, the less likely you would be to get stomach or gastrointestinal cancer. They found one such food: garlic!

In this research, other things in food, such as carotenoids, also reduce the risk of cancer, so they have to be factored out. After all the other factors were eliminated, garlic emerged.

Future research will cross the t's and dot the i's of these findings. Epidemiology research moves in slow motion owing to the difficulty in sorting through the many dietary records and demographic records, then relating one to the other; and this research is being done in many countries, not only in China. Consequently, obtaining results takes time. As I write this, results supporting this hypothesis are being reported at scientific meetings.

But the fog has lifted, and we know where we stand. When the biochemistry is clear, research in animals supports it, and it's confirmed by epidemiology, only the most dedicated skeptic would reserve judgment. Add the scientific studies to 3,550 years of human experience and you've got a compelling reason to use garlic in your cooking. Indeed, I think you've got an argument to use lots of garlic with the food you eat.

WORMS, PARASITES, AND BAD WATER

Garlic gets rid of worms and intestinal parasites. What might be called a national policy, using garlic was set in motion by Dioscorides, chief physician of the Roman army. Dioscorides used garlic to eliminate and prevent intestinal worms. His use of garlic found its way into the writings of Pliny, who is often mistakenly credited with recognizing its use as an intestinal vermifuge. A vermifuge is a material that eliminates vermin; in this case, worms and other intestinal parasites. Though this is not a problem in the United States, it's a strong reason to eat garlic when visiting third-world countries.

ONIONS AND GARLIC STOP DIABETES

People with diabetes have always claimed that onions reduce blood sugar. This was dismissed as another old wives' tale. When Dr. Kohrana Agusti saw so many patients who claimed it worked, he decided to put it to a clinical test. First, let me help you understand diabetes.

Diabetes is a condition in which the level of blood sugar or glucose is elevated, often to a dangerous level. This happens for two common reasons. The pancreas, a gland near the stomach, doesn't produce any insulin, or it doesn't produce enough insulin. If the pancreas can't make any insulin, we say the person has Type-I, or juvenile, diabetes because this type usually appears before the age of twenty. The only help is daily injections of insulin. Type-I diabetes seems to be a genetically inherited disease, but there is evidence that it's also diet-related through an immune problem. However, eating all the onions in the world won't solve Type-I diabetes.

Type-II, or adult-onset, diabetes develops as people get older. About 75 percent is triggered by being overweight. Weight reduction usually solves the problem and the blood sugar returns to normal. However, much adult-onset diabetes persists beyond weight loss because the pancreas simply doesn't produce enough insulin. Here's where onions help.

Agusti and his colleagues first gave adult-onset diabetics lots of onions. Their blood sugar became normal, as folklore claimed it would. Then Agusti's group tested onion oils that were taken from pressing onions and found that they also worked at normalizing blood sugar.

Another team, Doctors Gupta and Gupta, continued the research and tested extracts of onion oil against the standard drug tolbutamide, which is used to stimulate insulin production and lower blood sugar. On a comparative basis, the Gupta onion extract has about 80 percent of the tolbutamide activity with no side effects.

Therefore, the folklore is correct if you put it in perspective. Onions won't help a diabetic who must use insulin. If diabetes is caused by overweight, the thing to do is go on a diet. But beyond that, eat lots of onions, control your weight, and there's a good chance diabetes can be controlled without the use of drugs.

VAMPIRES

Everyone dismisses garlic's ability to ward off vampires as pure Hollywood hype. They're right about movie vampires, but not the legend that's behind it, which developed from a disease, porphyria, in which the blood is exceptionally sensitive to light; similar to the disease Dr. Mathews-Roth worked with (see chapter 1).

Porphyria is a hereditary disease that, in the past, occurred in isolated areas of central Europe, especially Rumania, where Transylvania, the land of vampires, is located. People with porphyria need iron in the form of hemoglobin from blood. They must avoid sunlight or any strong indoor light, lest they have a very severe skin reaction. This reaction causes their skin to become inflamed, painful, and produce toxins that make them very sick. They are exceptionally hairy, have large teeth, and very light skin. Sound like a vampire? This is how the vampire legend started. Most importantly, diallylsulfides make them violently ill. Allicin is the most common, naturally occurring diallylsulfide, and garlic is the best source. Therefore, if you're a victim of this hereditary porphyria, you'll look and act like a vampire and will avoid garlic like a deadbeat avoids bill collectors!

Bram Stoker must have done a lot of research on this for his famous novel. Even Hollywood got the folklore correct!

ONIONS, LEEKS, AND CHIVES

Most of what has been said about garlic also goes for onions, leeks, and other members of the botanical family, including asparagus. They all contain some allicin and its analogues to a lesser extent than garlic, so they aren't as effective, but they contribute to the whole effect.

Try to see your diet as an ongoing part of life that can make it better, last longer, and be more abundant. In this context, everything you eat adds or detracts from life's quality and quantity. So it's important not to focus only on garlic, but to see it as a major contributing factor and these other vegetables as secondary contributors. In that way, you can add chives to the sour cream on your potatoes, put a slice of onion on your salad, and add a crushed garlic clove to your pot of soup.

SAFETY

Garlic, onions, leeks, and shallots can be irritating to the skin of some people. Onions irritate the eyes of most people.

The lacrimatory (tear-producing) factor of onions has been the subject of research to find natural materials that will drive off an animal, such as a dog, without causing permanent injury. These factors in onions irritate the eyes naturally and prevent some animals from eating onions. Cut raw onions under water, as the irritating factors dissolve in water, and you'll never notice them.

Some people are sensitive to one or all of these bulbs. They itch, their skin gets red, and they have symptoms of contact dermatitis, similar to the rashes some people get from household solvents and detergents. Common sense dictates that if you're sensitive, you should stay away from these bulbs.

On the other extreme, certain people are allergic to one or more of these foods. Anyone with a food allergy knows enough to stay away from the food that causes it.

In clinical studies, researchers experimented with garlic or onion extracts. You, as a layperson, shouldn't do that. In telling you about these studies, I want to get you to use more of these bulbs as food. That's what they are and that's how they should be used.

DO GARLIC TABLETS WORK?

Experts tell me that kyolic garlic sold as tablets in health-food stores works as well as garlic. It is actually aged garlic pressed into tablets. My gut feeling tells me it's okay to use and just as effective as fresh. At the first international meeting on garlic, papers were presented to show that aged, kyolic garlic has the same properties as fresh, raw, garlic bulbs.

However, I'm skeptical about artificially deodorized garlic tablets. Some active components have the pungent, garlic odor, so it seems that if the odor is extracted by solvents, the effectiveness is lost. I still prefer to use fresh garlic, onions, leeks, chives, and asparagus.

PUTTING THIS KNOWLEDGE INTO FOOD

Did you know that baked garlic is nowhere near as pungent as fresh garlic, or that you can eat raw garlic cloves or even swallow small ones whole? For most people, a few rules will help you increase the protective benefit this marvelous plant affords.

MODERN FOLKLORE

A half clove of garlic a day keeps the doctor away. A whole clove does a better job. Half an onion a day helps.

SOME GARLIC DO's

- Add a clove of garlic to each serving of soup.
- Add a clove of garlic to a garden salad.
- Add a clove of garlic for each serving of fish, roast, or fowl.

- Add a half clove of garlic for each serving of spaghetti sauce, whether red or white.

- An omelet without garlic is like a day without sunshine.

GARLIC DON'Ts

- Don't use garlic salt; it's salt.

- Don't use deodorized garlic.

- Don't use garlic oil except in a recipe.

- Don't let a day pass without some garlic.

14

Cruciferous Vegetables

At the dawning of the Christian era, some Roman communities banned physicians from practicing and declared people could stay healthy by eating cabbage. Although medicine was primitive in A.D. 1, I'm not sure I would have dropped it in favor of cabbage, even if my mother did feed it to me whenever I was sick. Cabbage and other cruciferous vegetables, especially mustard, were always viewed as healthful foods and formed the basis of many home remedies.

By the way, cabbage is the oldest cultivated vegetable. Different varieties of cabbage grow wild in all parts of the world and have been cultivated by every agricultural society.

Cruciferous Vegetable Quiz

Answer yes or no to the following questions:

- Can you name five cruciferous vegetables?

- Do you know why boiling brussels sprouts will tarnish silver?

- Have you ever heard that a mustard plaster can get rid of a cold? Bronchitis? Pleurisy?

- If eating broccoli, brussels sprouts, or radishes every day would help prevent cancer, would you do it?

If you didn't answer yes to all these questions, you should read on and learn more about the cruciferous vegetables.

FOLK REMEDIES

All cruciferous vegetables produce a number of sulfur-containing materials, the thiocyanates. As these foods are cooked or simply allowed to stand, these sulfur compounds change. As they change, they release materials that will tarnish silver, smell "musty," and even taste bitter or pungent. Since you can't separate the senses of smell and taste while eating, one unpleasant sensation will dominate your reaction. That explains why some people, including President Bush, can't be faulted for what their taste buds or odor-sensing nerves tell them.

The mustard oil produced by all these cruciferous plants is used in various forms for medicinal purposes. One, the mustard plaster, was made of powdered mustard seed. When the powder is mixed with water the chemical reaction produces heat and releases aromatic materials that smell "important" and help to relieve nasal congestion. The mustard plaster could generate enough heat to blister the skin if a substantial layer of cloth wasn't placed between the plaster and the skin. The objective of the plaster was to localize heat in the chest. This heat helped stimulate circulation and loosen congestion, while the inhaled vapors from the oil attacked the congestion from the inside. Before the age of modern medicine, the mustard plaster was one of the most effective remedies available for easing if not curing bronchitis and pleurisy.

Mothers probably recognized certain characteristics in this type of plants, and their logic said: "If these plants could produce healing powers, they must be good to eat." Unfortunately, the same components that made them medicinal and tarnish silver also made some folks turn up their noses at them.

CRUCIFEROUS: THE CROSS

Cruciferous comes from the words *to crucify* or *to place on a cross*. The reproductive apparatus of cruciferous plants' flowers contains two components that can be arranged like a cross. This consistent characteristic lets scientists distinguish them from all other plants. Since most of us don't ever see their flowers, the name is important to botanists. Our objective is to simply eat the vegetable.

Once when I spoke on nutrition research, a mother proposed an experiment to save money spent on research. Her proposal was simple: Put a platter with a variety of plainly cooked vegetables on the table and take note of those the children eat least. They will be the most healthful vegetables. Her point was that children seem to have a natural aversion to the foods that are best for them. Surveys prove that children like brussels sprouts least, with cabbage and broccoli a close second and third in this negative contest. In contrast, epidemiologists place brussels sprouts, cabbage, and all the other cruciferous vegetables at the top of a list of plants known to prevent cancer. Score another point for mothers' common sense.

When President George Bush declared his dislike of broccoli, he supported these legions of young people who rank broccoli in the bottom three of their list. While we can appreciate a president's honesty, he didn't help further the aims of preventive medicine. Even though his taste buds may be sensitive to the unappetizing and odorous materials broccoli contains, there are ways of serving broccoli that make it quite delicious.

Epidemiologists who compare food habits of people who get cancer to those who don't notice a clear difference. People who eat cruciferous vegetables regularly have a much lower risk of many cancers, including cancers of the esophagus, stomach, colon, pancreas, lungs, breast, and skin.

This listing has no specific pattern and is what we'd expect if the protective factors were general to all tissues of the body. It seems to me that, if you go no further, having an extra serving of coleslaw, snacking on radishes, or eating bok choy or brussels sprouts is sensible eating.

Look at the list of common cruciferous vegetables and you'll agree there's plenty to choose from. And they are all protective.

TABLE 14.1

Cruciferous Vegetables

Broccoflower™	Japanese horseradish
Broccoli	Kale
Brussels sprouts	Kohlrabi
Cabbage (red, white, and others)	Mustard
Cauliflower	Radish
Chinese cabbage (bok choy)	Rutabaga
Cress	Turnip
Horseradish	Watercress

Fifteen common cruciferous vegetables are listed in table 14.1. I couldn't list every variety as there are over three thousand cruciferous plants, with many varieties in each group. For instance, there are over five varieties of cabbage and over twenty varieties of radishes readily available in the United States alone. Cruciferous vegetables are raised in every part of the world where the climate permits green plants to grow. Each agricultural area has its own unique varieties.

A STARTING POINT

Green tea and cabbage showed up together in epidemiology as being protective against cancer. Since they are botanically unrelated, people doing the research asked: "What does green tea have in common with cabbage?" Chemists answered quickly, "Phenols and indoles."

The common chemicals formed the link that gave scientists an idea of where to direct future research. So what has been an important ritual for over two thousand years in Japan has had a powerful protective effect in addition to its social value. The same is true for radishes, which are cruciferous vegetables, and are an important part of traditional Japanese meals.

This poses a dilemma for scientists who are trying to determine the relative protective value of these natural materials. You can't go up to someone and ask, "How many phenols, indoles, or isothiocyanates did you get in your food today?" Or, "How much sinigrin?'' While these materials are present in all cruciferous vegetables, the exact amounts vary widely, and the amount in each vegetable is generally unknown. Like any natural foods, their composition differs by variety, location grown, climate, rainfall, and soil conditions. At first scientists thought these substances were just another group of antioxidants, but they quickly realized there was something else going on. Soon it dawned on them that they had opened up a new horizon in protection. I'll explain this new type of protection by telling you how the discovery was made.

When epidemiologists noticed that bok choy and other cruciferous vegetables protect people from colon cancer, biochemists did follow-up studies on rats. First, they fed rats a well-understood chemical agent that causes colon cancer to see if bok choy is protective, as the epidemiologists said it was. And it was. The next step was to test other cruciferous vegetables and remove chemicals from them to see which chemicals are protective.

Animal testing has proven that indoles, phenols, flavons, thiocyanates, and a few other components from all cruciferous vegetables are protective. Once the factors were reduced to some chemicals, biochemists explored how these chemicals prevent cancer. Several findings emerged from the research that help us understand why these vegetables are so protective.

ANTIOXIDANTS AGAIN

The active, naturally occurring chemicals in the cruciferous vegetables and green tea are all antioxidants. If a chemist feeds an animal a combination of materials that produce antioxidants and free radicals, the results will show that, by themselves, these antioxidants will neutralize the free radicals. These results prove that the antioxidants from cruciferous vegetables by themselves protect us from cancer. In this regard, they act in the same way as vitamins E and C and the carotenoids.

The cruciferous vegetables are so consistently protective against cancer that biochemists studied them in much more detail than in just the free-radical experiments. These studies have opened up a new horizon that is more important than their antioxidant qualities. To understand what the materials in cruciferous vegetables do, I've got to digress and explain your body's enzymes.

ENZYMES MAKE LIVING THINGS UNIQUE

A large, modern chemical factory works with only a few processes, usually at high temperatures measured in hundreds of degrees. You'd fry at the temperatures they use. Your car engine is a small chemical processing factory that you use regularly. In the engine, gasoline is converted to carbon dioxide and water, while releasing the chemical energy stored in gasoline to run your car. Engine temperatures reach hundreds of degrees. Indeed, your car engine needs an elaborate cooling system so the engine doesn't burn up and so you can get close to it. Your body uses exactly the same process as your car engine to get energy from fats. Fats are so similar to gasoline that you could say it's just a variant and vice versa. However, your body gets more energy out of an ounce of fat than your car engine gets from an ounce of gasoline. In engineering terms, your body is more efficient. You might ask: Why isn't my body running at several hundred degrees? The answer is because your body's processes use enzymes.

Enzymes are proteins that our body makes to carry out its chemical processes. Sticking to your car engine example, enzymes make the same energy-yielding process take place in your body as in your car engine, but enzymes do it at body temperature. Your body extracts more energy, ounce for ounce, than your engine does, and produces exactly the same waste materials, carbon dioxide and water. The enzymes act as catalysts, which make the process occur rapidly at body temperatures, but aren't changed themselves in the process. In fact, enzymes are ready to process another batch of fat when the first one is done.

INDUCED PROTECTIVE ENZYMES

Biochemists who examined how body cells reacted to cruciferous vegetables were surprised. The cells produced new protective enzymes. I call them protective because they cause destruction of the free radicals, superoxides, and other materials that irritate cells and cause them to become dysplastic. These enzymes give the materials from cruciferous vegetables a second, unique role. Cruciferous vegetables cause each living cell to upgrade its own protective enzyme systems. This is a new concept in protection.

The process in which the number of enzymes increases as a result of an outside influence is known as enzyme induction. It means that the body cells make more of a particular enzyme in response to materials called inducers. In this case, inducers come from cruciferous vegetables. There may have been none or just a trace of a particular enzyme before the cruciferous vegetables came along. After you eat the vegetables and absorb their material, your body cells start to produce a lot of that enzyme. I guess we could call cruciferous vegetables "protective inducers," because they induce the cells to make protective enzymes.

It's important to know that our body couldn't make these enzymes if the plans to make them, the genetic code, weren't already locked into our genetic pool. Therefore, the need for them was anticipated by our maker. The induced protective enzymes fall into two classes: transferases and oxygenases. Transferases transfer a toxic material to something else, such as beta carotene, vitamin E, an indole, or some other antioxidant you got from a vegetable or fruit. An oxygenase simply causes toxic forms of oxygen to be broken down in a way that's not destructive. In both cases the toxin is neutralized. The "ase" on the end of a word signals that it's an enzyme if you're talking about a living system.

Superoxide dismutase is one of the enzymes that our body produces in response to eating cruciferous vegetables. As its name implies, superoxide dismutase breaks the toxic superoxide into pieces that are neutralized by other antioxidants such as the carotenoids, vitamin E, indoles, and other antioxidants from vegetables, including the cruciferous vegetables. Research in this area is very active since it gives us insight into how the body shores up its defenses against toxic agents.

The bottom line is clear. The cruciferous vegetables cause our body to boost its protective systems in a way we couldn't have predicted. They work like this: Materials in cruciferous vegetables signal each cell of the body to build more of its protective enzymes, for example, superoxide dismutase. Because the enzymes transfer toxic oxides to these antioxidant materials from cruciferous vegetables, cruciferous vegetables act as a signal—a switch—that turns protective enzyme production. And it boosts your protective power.

Importantly, some of the toxic materials that are neutralized are those that attack genetic material in the nucleus of all body cells. This fact provides the biochemical basis for the scientific observation that cruciferous vegetables seem to reduce the risk of all types of cancer. Though the protective effect is most obvious in the high-risk cancers that are most studied, such as colon, breast, and lung cancer, it's also observed in stomach, esophagus, pancreatic, and other lesser known cancers. This is exactly what you'd expect from foods that have such broad effects—signaling every cell in the body. As we study more cancers, I expect the protection by cruciferous vegetables to be almost universal.

I like to think of antioxidants and enzyme induction as the ultimate form of protection. Once the materials of protection are available, the body makes its own enzymes and uses them effectively. These enzymes go even further and use materials from the cruciferous vegetables to neutralize toxins. Our body then discards the neutralized toxins and is ready to take on more. To take advantage of this marvelous process, only one thing is asked of us, that we eat cruciferous vegetables regularly! How simple can our task be?

PROTECTION BEYOND CANCER

Even though you think "cancer's enough," there's more. Cancer is the second leading cause of death, which is one reason scientists are working so hard on its "cure." Other diseases aren't known as well because they aren't studied as extensively. They aren't as economically important, for one thing. What other diseases would be affected by the protection found in cruciferous vegetables?

Emphysema, unlike lung cancer, builds slowly. It isn't an "all or none" disease; it's not usually diagnosed until it's so bad it's obvious. Because emphysema can be caused by the same airborne toxins that cause lung cancer, any antioxidant that helps prevent lung cancer helps prevent emphysema. Therefore, cruciferous vegetables can protect us from emphysema. But emphysema is an obvious disease to relate to cruciferous vegetables. What else should we look at?

Cruciferous vegetables should play a prime role in neutralizing intestinal irritants, because their protection occurs throughout the body and because research has shown their protective effect in stomach and esophagus cancers. Therefore, we should find them associated with a reduced risk of ulcers and hemorrhoids, and we do. In fact, cabbage juice is a folk remedy for stomach ulcers. We don't know how it works in reality, but conceptually, it causes the stomach to build its own defenses.

Other effects from the materials in cruciferous vegetables relate to their ability to protect the integrity of the genetic materials. Keeping genetic material unchanged reduces the likelihood of defects that emerge during and after birth. In the future, materials from cruciferous vegetables will surely show up as being protective against all health problems where toxins are involved.

If I had to summarize, in a few words, what insights we've gained from the biochemistry between us and the cruciferous vegetables, I'd say: "It has opened the door that hides the secret of aging, because all these observations are expressions of the aging process." Indeed, skin wrinkles, cataracts, and deteriorating tissues result from free radical attack. The more we diffuse these natural explosives, the slower the aging process will occur.

GETTING CRUCIFEROUS VEGETABLES

- Each day have at least one serving of a cruciferous vegetable.

- Eat three varieties of cruciferous vegetables a week.

- Eat one serving raw twice weekly; for example, cabbage or radishes.

PART

IV

THE LONGEVITY PROGRAM

In the very few minutes it takes to read this page, about five people in the United States will die of either cancer or heart diseases. Correct diet could have prevented their deaths or at least delayed them for many years. These people could have enjoyed the abundance of life much longer.

Life expectancy has many determinants. A girl born today has a life expectancy of about seventy-nine years. If, by some miracle, we could prevent all causes of death before she reached age fifty, it would only increase her life expectancy by about three or four years. That's because, according to statistics, the vast majority of deaths occur after the age of fifty.

Another way of looking at life expectancy is to imagine everyone applying the knowledge we have about diet and health, if everyone followed the principles of the Longevity Diet in the next chapter, and used a good supplement plan. The reward would be reducing the risk of cancer and heart disease by over 50 percent. In short, if the newborn girl's parents put this dietary plan to work before she was conceived and raised her by its principles, and if it became her life-long eating habit, her life span could exceed the current expectancy by about 30 percent. She'd live past one hundred and three! And the quality of her life would be good for far longer; she'd be active and alert, not just alive.

If you add on the years continuing advances in medicine will contribute to the newborn girl's life, she could easily live for one hundred and fifteen or one hundred and twenty years. She'd be a cinch to celebrate New Year's Eve in A.D. 2100! In short, her life would span an entire century.

In the next two chapters, you'll learn the details of the Longevity Diet. I call it this because it increases your longevity. It puts the protectors on a daily basis. It lets you practice prevention whether you eat at home or in restaurants and even when you're enjoying some snacks. This diet combines the protectors and the balanced diet of good nutrition that you read about in the papers but seldom see spelled out. The objective of this diet can be summarized in this axiom: ''Nutrition is preventive medicine, and food is the vehicle of its practice.''

After you have looked at the Longevity Diet, the chapter that follows gives you some ideas for daily menus and includes some interesting and healthful tips about certain ethnic foods. I'll also give you a checklist to help you select food supplements. This array of choices will prove that the variety of ways you can apply this plan are endless and, we hope, habit-forming.

15

The Longevity Diet
Don't Get Older,
Get Better

"Hold fast to the spirit of youth; let years come to what they may."
—Advice to young students at Columbia University

The Longevity Diet makes it easier to hold fast to the spirit of youth. It puts the protectors into everyday practice and is balanced by all the criteria for good health. Follow it faithfully and your physiological age will continue to fall behind your chronological age. If you feel "old" now, give it time, and you'll feel younger.

If you follow the Longevity Diet, I promise that within a week you will feel better than you do now. You'll sleep more soundly at night and get up with more bounce in the morning. Within a month, you'll look better, and people will notice it. Stick with the diet plan and your risks of cancer and heart diseases will decline in proportion to the length of time you follow the diet.

Other minor and, depending on your point of view, possibly more important benefits will accrue. Your skin won't wrinkle as quickly. You'll recover from minor ailments faster. You'll have more energy and be more alert mentally. If you're overweight, you'll drop the extra pounds. Add exercise, and you'll convert body fat to muscle. You'll be pleased with the "new you."

Many people live to eat. I want you to learn to eat to live. Anyone can follow the Longevity Diet. It's endless in variety—no two meals or snacks have to be the same. Once you work this diet plan into your lifestyle, it becomes habit; the best habit you'll ever develop!

THE LONGEVITY DIET

Protective Eating

1. Fruits and Vegetables: 5 Servings Daily

Vegetables: ½ cup cooked or 1 cup raw.
Examples: A single, large stalk of broccoli with the florets; 6 medium asparagus spears; 2 cooked potatoes without skin or 1 baked potato with skin; 1 cup cooked white or wild rice; 1 medium-sized raw carrot.

Fruit: A medium apple, orange, pear, or similar fruit; 3 small plums or apricots; ⅛ a large cantaloupe; half a small melon; a 1-inch slice of watermelon.

Four Rules Apply:

- Eat one serving of deep green or dark red vegetables, such as spinach, broccoli, sweet red pepper, carrots.

- Eat one serving of fruit raw, such as an orange, apple, banana.

- Eat three servings of beans weekly, such as lima, red kidney, lentils. Change varieties regularly.

- Eat one serving of a mixed salad with tomatoes and onions.

2. Grains and Cereals: 4 Servings Daily

Cereals: ⅓ cup cold or cooked; emphasize cereals that provide 4 or more grams of fiber per serving.

Breads: 1 slice whole-grain bread or 1 whole-grain roll.

Pasta: 1 cup cooked; 2 ounces dry.

Grains: ½ cup cooked.
- One daily serving high-fiber, natural cereal with low-fat or

non-fat milk. Try to eat three varieties of high-fiber cereals weekly.

3. Natural Bulbs: 1 Serving Daily

A serving of natural bulbs is not as precise a measurement as it is for other vegetables. Eat garlic, onions, leeks, shallots, and chives regularly.

Examples: 1 clove of garlic to flavor a salad, soup, meat, spaghetti sauce, etc.; ¼ onion in your salad or with some vegetables; ¼ cup chopped raw leeks. Flavor foods with these bulbs regularly. You can't get too much.

4. Milk and Dairy Products: 3 Low-Fat Servings Daily

Milk: One cup.

Yogurt: 6 ounces.

Cheese: About 1½ ounces or 40 grams.

- Although ice cream is a dairy product, it requires 1 full pint to fulfill the nutritional need. Frozen yogurt is somewhat better, because it contains fewer calories, but it still calls for 1 pint. Newer low-fat ice creams are better yet.

5. Protein-Rich Foods: 2 Servings Daily

Fish, fowl, meat: 3½ ounces (about ¼ pound).

Eggs: 2 medium.

Cheese: 1½ ounces.

Beans: 1 cup cooked.

Weekly Rules to Follow:

- Eat fish at least 3 times; fin fish at least twice.

- Eat 1 vegetarian meal; for example, pasta with cheese; eggs; beans.

- Eat fowl as often as desired; remove the skin after cooking.

- Eat red meat only once a week.

- Don't eat processed meats, such as bologna, hot dogs, and so on.

6. Oils and Fats

Frying: Peanut oil, olive oil, or butter. Don't use canola or other oil high in polyunsaturated fats.

Baking: Canola oil, rapeseed oil.

Salads: Olive, canola, walnut, avocado, linseed oils.

Additive: Add 1 teaspoon flaxseed oil daily to salad dressing and in baking to increase the omega-3 oils.

7. Water

Drink four 8-ounce glasses daily. Use purified water, mineral-water, or distilled water. Seek out water that is free of nitrates, chlorides, and manmade chemicals, such as pesticides. Natural minerals, including calcium, magnesium, and so on, should be prized.

To determine food alternatives, the following source book is recommended:

Bowes & Church's
Food Values of Portions Commonly Used
Jean A. T. Pennington, Ph.D., R.D.
15th Edition, 1989
J. B. Lippincott, Philadelphia

I encourage you to go beyond this diet. If you become a fish-eating almost-vegetarian in contrast to the typical meat-eating American who eats 6.5 ounces of beef daily, you'll accelerate the benefits of the diet and will live better sooner.

Think of your body as a castle and the Longevity Diet as its foundation. Although scientists will argue over the value of megadosing on vitamins and minerals, there's unanimous agreement on applying the principles of the diet with a heavier hand than the basics. A few easy additions will pay dividends. For example:

- Up to nine servings of fruits and vegetables daily are better than the basic five.

- Eating fish four or five times weekly is better than three; and no red meat is even better than some.

- Extra cruciferous vegetables and foods from the garlic family will add to the benefits. It's a true case of more is better.

- A high-fiber bran cereal is an excellent start for every day. Oat bran, wheat bran, rice bran, or corn bran are excellent for variety.

- An extra serving of beans prepared without fat will help reduce cholesterol and the risk of all the illnesses I've discussed.

- Sensible supplementation will help.

A few habits can make the Longevity Diet even more effective. You've heard them before, but they're worth repeating.

- Eat fruit for dessert. For example, a slice of melon, half a mango, or a slice of watermelon. Fruit is cheaper in the long run than traditional desserts and provides all the protectors.

- Snack on vegetables, fruit, and nuts. They all provide protectors.

- Always use whole grain breads or rolls.

- Drink an 8-ounce glass of water first thing in the morning, 30 minutes before each meal, and once before bedtime.

If you follow the Longevity Diet, you'll get enough fiber, carotenoids, bioflavonoids, folic acid, and the other things from food that protect your health. However, the level of some nutrients, such as vitamins E, C, and others, are more protective when you get them in higher amounts than diet can provide. Therefore, it's fair for you to ask: "Are the RDAs enough?" and "Do I need supplements?"

RDA VERSUS PROTECTOR NEED

Vitamins C and E are called for at higher levels as protectors than as basic nutrients, the case in which their RDA requirement applies to them. The higher level is needed for the protector purpose because vitamins C and E act differently as vitamins and as protectors. As vitamins, they can be reused by your body with only minute amounts lost in each use. As protectors they actually neutralize toxins and are destroyed in the process. The protector function is not always the same as the vitamin function. For the same reason, we also need more protective beta carotene than is required to make vitamin A. There's no RDA for tocopherols besides alpha tocopherol, for carotenoids like lycopene, or for other nutrients, such as fiber, so the protector function should be the criterion of need. The concepts here are not at odds with the RDAs.

At the risk of repetition, let me say again that RDAs are designed for satisfactory health and protection from deficiency symptoms. They achieve both objectives with flying colors. Our society is free of identifiable deficiency diseases, and two levels of safety are satisfied.

RDAs have about a 40-percent low-end safety factor built into them. This means that if you get only 60 percent of the RDA, you'll be generally free of nutritional deficiency symptoms. By government standards, you'll be in satisfactory health, and that's as it should be.

If you exceed the RDA, say up to over ten times the amount specified, with two exceptions, you'll be free of toxicity symptoms. The two exceptions, which aren't completely clear, are vitamins A and D. Don't confuse beta carotene or other carotenoids with vitamin A. Beta carotene is only converted to vitamin A as required, so there's no beta carotene overdose. You can't get toxic levels of vitamin D from sunshine, because your body has the built-in safety of its skin pigments. If you use vitamin-D-fortified dairy products or calcium supplements, you'll be safe. There's a natural safety and regulated safety associated with vitamins A and D. It takes serious abuse of vitamin-A and vitamin-D supplements, usually coupled with ignorance, for a toxic situation to develop. Use common sense.

When the RDAs were determined, protector functions were not taken into account. These protector functions have emerged because we live much longer, on average, than when scientists first started to assign nutritional need. In those days we didn't think of diseases, like cancer, cataracts, and emphysema, as dietary issues. And no one thought about neutralizing toxins, such as nitrates or excess ultraviolet light. Our longevity represents the triumphs of modern medicine. However, the protector function of nutrients and food components opens new horizons for nutritional biochemistry and personal responsibility.

DO YOU NEED SUPPLEMENTS?

As the twentieth century winds down, we find that sensible use of supplements can help everyone. Compare supplements to pocket calculators. It's good to be able to calculate square roots by long-hand, but it's a more efficient use of your time to use the calculator. Supplements are a little like that. They don't substitute for the Longevity Diet; they make it better. Diet will always be the foundation of health; supplements strengthen that foundation a little bit more.

A survey of registered dieticians by the American Dietetic Association revealed that about 55 percent of them use food supplements. That's 10 percent more than the 45 percent of average folks who use them. Dieticians are the same people who say you can get what you need from a balanced diet. Although it sounds a little like the doctor who says to stop smoking while he lights up a cigarette, it isn't. It proves that the experts want to insure the balanced diet they try and follow, or that they realize that stresses in our complex world impose greater nutrient demands on our bodies than food alone can satisfy. They're also more aware of the protective power some nutrients provide, and they simply want to "hedge their bets." Supplements are an insurance policy for them and should be the same for you. I've included a list of basic, general supplements that will insure that your basic nutrition won't be lacking.

Multivitamin-Multimineral Supplements

Supplement	Company	Comments Per Tablet
Vita-Lea	Shaklee Corporation	50% U.S. RDA Calcium 30% Magnesium 25%
Centrum	Lederle	100% U.S. RDA Calcium 16% Magnesium 25%
Theragran M	E. R. Squibb and Sons	100% U.S. RDA Calcium 4% Magnesium 25%
Myadec	Parke Davis	100% U.S. RDA Calcium 7% Magnesium 25%
Geritol Complete	Beechum Products	100% U.S. RDA Calcium 16% Magnesium 25%
Multi-Essentials	MXM Essential Formulas	100% RDA Calcium 7% Magnesium 5%

In earlier chapters I discussed other supplements, such as beta carotene, fiber, vitamin C, calcium, and B-complex. In the next chapter I give a brief checklist for other supplements. You must assess your own diet against the Longevity Diet and what you've read here to see if you need more.

SUPPLEMENTS: MISCONCEPTIONS

When I speak to people here and abroad about nutrition, I'm amazed by two very different groups of people who have misconceptions about nutrition for the same reasons. One group takes large amounts or megadoses of food supplements. It's not uncommon for someone to tell me he takes 5 grams of vitamin C daily or as many as ten to twenty different supplements. The other group's members have usually tried supplements but couldn't see a difference in how they felt, so they stopped. I find that neither group is particularly careful or expert about their diet.

Megavitamin abusers think that vitamin supplements can make up for not eating a good diet. They try and separate food from nutrition. In short, they get pleasure from food and seek nutrition from pills. Many of these people think they can eat anything as long as they take copious quantities of supplements. I've noticed that they are often seriously overweight.

In contrast to the megavitamin abusers are the people who think that if they take supplements today, tomorrow they'll be able to leap buildings in a single bound like Superman. These people expect to get the same quick results that a strong drug, prescribed for an illness, delivers. These people often have a poor attitude about diet, too. Because they don't notice the effects of diet or supplements quickly, they usually don't bother taking either their diet or their supplements seriously. They lose out in two ways.

ARE MEGADOSES THE ANSWER?

Chapter 2 pointed out the value of taking some extra vitamin C in addition to eating more fruit, vegetables, and cereals. While statistics show that 320 milligrams of vitamin C daily is a cutoff that reduces the risk of breast cancer, they also show that your odds improve with about 25 milligrams of beta carotene, 30 grams of fiber, about 60 micrograms of selenium, and regular exercise. So taking an extra 500 milligrams of vitamin C is an important risk reducer, in my opinion, but other nutrients are needed as well. This is a good example of the need for a total commitment.

Nutrition is far from being an exact science. There are factors in food, such as the flavonoids and the factors in cruciferous vegetables, that seem to make vitamin C more effective or that can replace it altogether. Similarly, there are about three hundred and fifty other carotenoids in foods besides beta carotene. The roles of these factors are not well understood, but they're probably important; we just don't know how their effects accumulate. Therefore, taking extra vitamin C in pill form will certainly do some good, but eating an extra orange or kiwi fruit might enhance its results even more.

NUTRITION IS A SLOW-MOTION TONIC

Unless you have a serious, diet-related, health problem, you won't detect a significant physical change overnight from the Longevity Diet, even if you use additional supplements. Improving your nutrition always pays, but the most powerful dividends, such as a longer life, accumulate slowly without notice. Nutrition is about wellness, not illness.

An aggressive program of self-health renewal includes attention to diet, lifestyle, and sensible food supplements. Any person who wants to see how well the Longevity Diet works should keep a personal health diary for a month or two, recording daily how they feel, look, sleep, and wake up, and their energy level, regularity, and disposition. If you keep a diary like this you won't be disappointed because you'll see results. A health diary is a good way to get in touch with your body and understand your feelings—you'll discover the best "you."

For example, people who follow a diet plan to lower blood pressure usually detect significant results in a week or ten days. And in four to eight weeks, many can stop using medication. In contrast, when people follow a dietary program to help arthritis, they usually get some results in ten days and mild results in about three or four weeks, but it requires six months for obvious improvements in mobility, inflammation, and pain. Even then, a person with arthritis can seldom stop taking some form of medication at least occasionally. People who follow the Longevity Diet and add supplements can identify subtle but definite results within a few days, even though the diet is a lifetime commitment. For example, in a week or two your fingernails usually become a little stronger with a healthy, pink color beneath the nail bed, all of which reflect better metabolism and circulation. People also notice within a few days that they sleep more soundly and wake up with more energy. In about a week, stamina improves and they feel more relaxed while having as much energy at the end of the day as at the beginning.

These changes are indications of better general health. They are subtle and accumulate so slowly that most people are unaware of them. What's worse, if you stop your nutrition commitment, the benefits will decline as slowly as they started, so even when they go away, you don't notice them. You'll think it's normal.

Bowel regularity is the change that everyone experiences quickly. Government surveys show that most people consume less than 50 percent of the dietary fiber they need. Within a few days after following the Longevity Diet, people start to notice a change in their bowel movements; they'll have one every twenty-four to thirty-six hours. One couple said they stopped using a daily laxative. In addition to making you feel better, regularity also helps your complexion. By the way, the old saying ''An apple a day keeps the doctor away'' got started over eight hundred years ago from the good effects that regularity produces, the most obvious of which is a good complexion.

Your health evolved to its present state over many years. It's the sum total of heredity, environment, diet, lifestyle, and emotions, along with all your good and bad habits. Therefore, the fact that you can notice an effect from diet within a few weeks or a month is truly spectacular. It shows how your body responds to a little nutritional support.

WEIGHT AND BLOOD PRESSURE: TWO DIVIDENDS

Weight loss is a major American pastime. Over 26 percent of Americans are obese, being 20 percent or more above normal weight. At least once during the year most adults diet to lose 5 to 10 pounds and seldom succeed. Weight loss is one of our nation's largest industries and, in spite of all the money spent, we're still overweight. Heavy Americans seem to have soft, blubbery fat, while people from other nations may be heavy, but they appear more firm. Firmness has to do with activity.

Stanford Medical School worked for several years with several communities to reduce the risk factors of heart disease. They succeeded with smoking, blood pressure, cholesterol, and all the other risk factors they monitored, except weight loss. In spite of the efforts by a ''who's who'' group of experts, the community level of obesity didn't budge! Overweight is one of the most intractable of all health risks. It's a disease that doesn't lend itself to fast cures. It requires a *total* dietary commitment, not just a few weeks' worth.

If you follow the Longevity Diet, add on exercise, and use common sense to avoid empty calories, your weight will drop naturally but slowly. Weight loss happens on this plan because you'll be reducing the calories in your diet and increasing its bulk. It's the natural result of a low-fat, correct-fiber, high-carbohydrate diet. You'll feel full most of the time. Increase your exercise level and you will accelerate the process of weight improvement.

Another dividend of weight loss and the Longevity Diet is better blood pressure. Most high blood pressure results from simple overweight, excessive salt, inadequate potassium, poor fat balance, and not enough fiber, in that order. Next to overweight, high blood pressure is our nation's most common illness, affecting over 23 percent of all adults. What's worse is that it's becoming an increasing concern in children. Over 4.5 percent of people under age eighteen have high blood pressure. Even slightly high blood pressure causes evidence of heart disease by age fifteen. If you have borderline high blood pressure that your doctor calls "high normal," your life will be shortened. I recommend you take immediate control. My book *The High Blood Pressure Relief Diet* explains the origins of high blood pressure and how to reduce it by diet. It even contains tested recipes. The dietary plan is compatible with the Longevity Diet. One compliments the other, and you can eat all the protector foods and use the supplements.

I can't speak about good nutrition without including exercise. Exercise is one of the simplest and most positive lifestyle changes that anyone can make. Even if you exercise regularly, read on about the protective power of exercise.

PROTECTIVE EXERCISE

Aerobic exercise improves circulation and builds the capacity of your heart and lungs. We call this cardiovascular fitness. Aerobic exercise was made popular and pioneered by Dr. Kenneth Cooper, who founded the famous Aerobics Institute in Dallas, Texas. Dr. Cooper has done more research on exercise and has done more to extoll the virtues of exercise for everyone than any other expert in this field. He has applied exercise to weight loss, body fat, cholesterol, and blood pressure, so I urge you to purchase one of his excellent books for yourself.

Exercise is a protector. When you exercise steadily (a brisk, thirty- or forty-minute walk is enough), the temperature inside your muscles increases by about two and a half degrees. This temperature change increases your metabolic rate by 17 to 35 percent, depending on your physical condition and content of body fat.

You can easily detect this metabolic increase by the rise in your pulse rate. It might increase from sixty-five beats per minute to one hundred and thirty-five beats. Your heart rate increases as your heart sends more blood throughout your body to send more oxygen to all of your body tissues in order to satisfy the demands of increased metabolism. But there's another important process going on as well.

With the increased circulation and the metabolic rate increase of all tissues, more byproducts of metabolism are removed and eliminated. In addition, every gland and tissue gets a workout, so it causes all of them to eliminate wastes and be replenished.

I compare exercise to the renewal and the cleansing of streets that come with a steady, spring rain. The rain leaves everything clean and glistening, naturally renewed, especially the plants. That's what exercise does for every cell, gland, and tissue in your body. Each exercise session leaves it renewed.

Many studies have proven that regular exercise reduces the risk of cancer, heart disease, high blood pressure, and even improves mental disorders. Exercise increases self-confidence and produces a positive outlook. When exercise is good, the brain produces low levels of natural opiates that actually improve your mental outlook. So, not only are you physically better, you also feel that way as well. There's one catch: exercise has to be sensible and regular for these benefits to develop.

In contrast to regular, moderate exercise, people who in a burst of enthusiasm go for broke and try to regain their vigor all at once do more harm than good. A good comparison is not the gentle, steady, spring rain that renews the flowers and cleans the streets, but the torrential downpour that wrecks houses, causes the sewage systems to overflow, kills plants and even people. It's a disaster.

Twenty to forty minutes of modest exercise, depending on activity level, five days a week is all it takes. That's about three hours weekly invested in better physical health, an improved outlook, better looks, and a longer life with more freedom from illness. Like a good diet, exercise is an investment that provides a 100-percent return.

I DON'T HAVE TIME

Talk of exercise brings the old excuse: "I don't have time." That's just a cop-out. In my career I've been a professor, have worked at every level in industry from the ground floor to the level of senior vice-president of a Fortune 500 company. My responsibilities covered several continents. I always find time for exercise by asking myself a very simple question: "What's more important than my health?"

One characteristic I've noticed in successful executives is an ability to set priorities. And when it comes to our personal life, we're the top executive. The buck stops with the face you see in the mirror! What priority in our life can be put above our health? I don't know of a single one. You don't have to be a Christian to appreciate Jesus, who said it simply: "Greater love has no man than he lay down his life for a friend." If the medium of exchange is love and our life is our most valued possession, doesn't it follow that personal health should be our number one priority? If you agree, you'll find time for exercise.

PUT THEORY INTO PRACTICE

Whenever I lecture on this diet, especially to medical students, I'm asked, "Do you follow this diet?" I answer yes. Then I'm asked, "How?" In the next chapter I've illustrated some menus that put this plan into daily reality. In addition, I've included an approximate calorie breakdown to prove you'll be eating better.

Let this diet become your eating habit and pass its concepts on to your loved ones. Their reward will be a longer and more abundant life. You will be putting an important axiom into practice: "Nutrition is preventive medicine and food is the vehicle of its practice."

16

The Longevity Diet Menus
One Day at a Time

"If I'd known I was going to need this body so long, I'd have started taking care of it a lot sooner."
—Satchel Paige, a baseball great

After I finished a lecture on dieting, a woman asked me, "When do I start?" "Immediately," I answered.

This first instant of the rest of your life is the best time to start developing habits that will help you live longer and live better. And if you're like me, you'd like a few examples to get started. This chapter will help you begin this worthwhile challenge.

MENUS: A GUIDELINE

I've used the Longevity Diet and each chapter in this book to develop seven daily food plans to illustrate the versatility of the diet. My objective is to stimulate your own creativity. Make a contest out of designing more imaginative and varied menus than mine. If you do, you are already on your way to a longer, healthier life. It's a contest where everyone is a winner.

SAMPLE MENUS FOR A WEEK

DAY 1

Meal	Calories

Breakfast

Glass of water	
½ grapefruit	39
All-Bran cereal	70
with low-fat milk (104), ½ sliced banana (52)	156
1 slice whole-grain bread, toasted (61) and buttered (36)	97
Tea or coffee, optional	

Mid-morning Snack

Glass of water	
Peach yogurt	260

Lunch

Glass of water	
Bean soup	157
1 whole-wheat roll (72) with butter (36)	108
Lettuce salad (4) with tomatoes (12), cucumber (4),	
green pepper (5), and onions (4), Italian dressing (14)	43
Lime sherbert	135
Tea or coffee, optional	

Afternoon Snack

Glass of water	
Apple (81) with cheddar cheese (114)	195

Dinner

Glass of water	
Broiled salmon with herbs	100
Baked potato (88) with sour cream and chives (26)	114
Steamed broccoli	12
Low-fat ice cream (140) with sliced strawberries (22)	162
Tea or coffee, optional	

Evening Snack

Pear	98

Day 1 Total	**1746**

DAY 2

Meal	Calories

Breakfast

Glass of water	
Slice of cantaloupe	57
Oatmeal (109) with raisins (56), low-fat milk (104)	269
Whole-wheat English muffin (170), butter (36)	206
Tea or coffee, optional	

Mid-morning Snack

Glass of water	
Bran muffin	112

Lunch

Glass of water	
Tuna fish salad (172) sandwich on whole-wheat bread (122)	294
Carrot sticks	31
Coleslaw	42
Tea or coffee, optional	

Afternoon Snack

Glass of water	
Pear (98) with feta cheese (75)	173

Dinner

Glass of water	
Cheese ravioli with tomato sauce with onions, garlic, spices	284
Mixed salad greens (5) with tomatoes (12), green pepper (5), garbanzo beans (32), Italian dressing (14)	68
Cannoli	171
Tea or coffee, optional	

Evening Snack

Apple	81

Day 2 Total	**1788**

DAY 3

Meal	Calories

Breakfast

Glass of water	
Orange-grapefruit juice	80
Sliced oranges and strawberries	55
Whole-wheat waffles (206) with maple syrup (50)	256
Tea or coffee, optional	

Mid-morning Snack

Glass of water	
Cheddar cheese (114) and grapes (75)	189

Lunch

Glass of water	
Salmon quiche	215
Triple-bean salad	90
Pear	98
Tea or coffee, optional	

Afternoon Snack

Glass of water	
Carrot and celery sticks	35

Dinner

Glass of water	
Wok chicken with broccoli, red peppers, onion, garlic, ginger, and mushrooms	266
Rice	112
Mixed green salad (5) with water chestnuts (15), green onions (7), and mandarin oranges (23), thousand island dressing (24)	74
Apple-tapioca pudding	101
Tea or coffee, optional	

Evening Snack

Banana	105

Day 3 Total	**1676**

DAY 4

Meal	Calories

Breakfast

Glass of water	
Slice of melon (57) with blueberries (41)	98
2 poached eggs (158) on whole-wheat toast (63)	221
1 slice lean ham	50
Tea or coffee, optional	

Mid-morning Snack

Glass of water	
Blueberry muffin	176

Lunch

Glass of water	
Curried chicken salad on lettuce	136
Banana bread	85
Frozen banana yogurt	143
Tea or coffee, optional	

Afternoon Snack

Glass of water	
Grapes	58

Dinner

Glass of water	
Halibut steak, broiled	119
Mixed green salad (5) with tomatoes (12), onions (7), red pepper (6), zesty tomato dressing (11)	38
Carrots	31
Asparagus	12
Rice	112
Apple strudel	96
Tea or coffee, optional	

Evening Snack

Brick cheese (105) and whole-wheat crackers (70)	175
Pear	98

Day 4 Total	**1648**

DAY 5

Meal	Calories

Breakfast

Glass of water   72
Sliced oranges, bananas, and kiwi fruit   164
Fiber One cereal (60) with low-fat milk (104)   148
Bran muffin (112), butter (36)
Tea or coffee, optional

Mid-morning Snack

Glass of water
Fruit yogurt   260

Lunch

Glass of water   69
Lentil soup   238
Melted cheese and crab on English muffin
Mixed salad greens (5) with tomatoes (12) and cucumbers (4),   32
     zesty tomato dressing (11)
Pear   98
Tea or coffee, optional

Afternoon Snack

Glass of water   59
Celery sticks (12) with peanut butter (47)   31
Carrot sticks

Dinner

Glass of water
Zucchini lasagne with tomato sauce with onions, garlic,   189
     and herbs   89
Corn   57
Lemon, cabbage, carrot mold with lettuce   81
Crusty French bread, butter   150
Cheesecake
Tea or coffee, optional

Evening Snack

Plum   36

Day 5 Total	1783

DAY 6

Meal	Calories

Breakfast

Glass of water
½ papaya | 59
Fiber One cereal (60) with low-fat milk (104) and blueberries (41) 205
Tea or coffee, optional

Mid-morning Snack

Glass of water
Fruit yogurt | 260

Lunch

Glass of water
Spinach salad with mushrooms, chopped egg, onion, bacon bits,
   oil, vinegar and mustard dressing | 218
Popover | 90
Sliced peaches | 66
Tea or coffee, optional

Afternoon Snack

Glass of water
Rice cakes (35) with cream cheese (98) | 133

Dinner

Glass of water
Filet of sole | 80
Basil bean salad with onions, garlic | 90
Rice pilaf | 121
Spinach | 6
Pumpkin pie | 212
Tea or coffee, optional

Evening Snack

Pear | 98

Day 6 Total   **1638**

DAY 7

Meal	Calories

Breakfast

Glass of water
Sliced peaches (37) with low-fat cottage cheese (41) 78
Whole-wheat pancakes (142) with blueberries (41) and
   maple syrup (50) 233
Tea or coffee, optional

Mid-morning Snack

Glass of water
Fruit yogurt 260

Lunch

Glass of water
Creamy carrot soup 149
Salmon salad with lettuce and tomato in pita bread 136
Raspberries 61
Tea or coffee, optional

Afternoon Snack

Glass of water
Applesauce wheat bar 134

Dinner

Glass of water
Marinated lamb roast with garlic 180
Tossed greens (5) with sliced canned pears (50) 55
Small roasted potatoes 65
Green beans 22
Whole-wheat roll with butter 70
Lemon dream parfaits 176
Tea or coffee, optional

Evening Snack

Orange 65

Day 7 Total	**1684**

CALORIES COUNT

As you look over the menu plan, you'll notice that each food item has its approximate calorie count, and the daily calories are totaled to show you that you won't get fat eating this way. In fact, I'll make a promise: If you're overweight now, and you start living by the Longevity Diet, your weight will slowly drop to normal.

However, this isn't a weight-loss plan. It's a healthful, sensible way of eating. Any weight loss comes because you're eating a more bulky diet with less fat and fewer simple carbohydrates (sugar). You'll feel full and won't get cravings.

HOW MANY CALORIES DO I NEED?

Placing calories alongside menus is good news for those who watch calories. It's bad news for those who don't, because natural curiosity raises a question: "How many calories do I need each day?"

Table 16.1 gives you an idea of how many calories you need, depending on how you spend your day. Most of us lead lives that are somewhere between sedentary and moderately active. I've put these two extremes of calorie balance together for you in table 16.1 so you can estimate your own needs.

TABLE 16.1

Daily Calorie Balance for Average People

Height	Weight	Age 30 Activity Level		Age 50 Activity Level	
		Sedentary	Moderately Active	Sedentary	Moderately Active
		Women			
5'2"	130	1750	2045	1660	1930
5'5"	145	1910	2225	1805	2105
5'7"	155	2020	2355	1910	2225

Men

5'10"	180	2385	2780	2270	2645
6'0"	190	2480	2890	2360	2760
6'2"	200	2600	3030	2470	2885

Calories are always approximate and were calculated as follows:
A. Basal metabolic rates (BMR) from body surface area charts
B. Activity Level
    Sedentary person: 0.2 times BMR
    Moderately active person: 0.4 times BMR
C. Calories lost to assimilation   0.1 times BMR + activity
    Total daily calories = A + B + C

Sedentary (mostly sitting): e.g., secretary, computer clerk
Moderately active: e.g., nurse, waiter or waitress
Most people fall between these two extremes. However, a carpenter (active) would be about 0.5 times BMR.
Exercise: If you exercise as recommended in this book, you will burn an additional 200 to 400 calories depending on your size, vigor of exercise, and time spent.

Just keep a few things in mind. We're all different, and we all use different amounts of energy for the same processes. In addition, we each digest and absorb our food a little differently. So, if two people follow this diet plan, one might lose a little weight and the other might stay the same. It's highly unlikely that anyone would gain weight, because this meal plan calls for a lot of bulk (fruit and vegetables) and is low in fat.

SERVING SIZE

In writing menu plans and preparing meals, nutritionists and dieticians use standard portions, such as ½ cup or 3.5 ounces, or practical portions, like one apple. This allows you to use standard food composition handbooks, recipe books, or nutritional labels on packaged foods to make your own meal plans. You can get an idea of how to adjust your serving size and substitute foods if gaining or losing weight is an objective. If you follow the plan and reduce your serving size, it can become the best weight-loss plan you'll ever follow.

Suppose a 6'4", 200-pound linebacker is married to a 5'4" fashion model who weighs 120 pounds. If they both eat the same meals according to this plan, adjusting serving sizes will keep him from shrinking and her from becoming huge. His servings will naturally be larger than hers. He might have two pears to her half pear or perhaps take a double serving of fish. The size of the portions doesn't matter, because the protector composition of the food is the same. Both partners are going to be as healthy as each other and still remain the unique individuals they are.

One more time: "Everyone who follows this plan is a winner."

SUPPLEMENTS

"What supplements should I use besides the basic supplement for nutritional insurance described in chapter 15?" "I read an article the other day that said vitamins are a waste of money." "My doctor said I can get everything from a balanced diet."

My intention is for you to make your own decision on supplements. If you decide for yourself, you'll be firm in your decision and won't need to be concerned with critics who advocate one side or the other.

BEYOND THE BASICS?

I believe the findings about certain nutrients are definitely in favor of taking them above and beyond what the Longevity Diet and a basic supplement provides. Consider the following:

- *Vitamin C:* If you take an additional 500 milligrams daily, you will have a sufficient excess of vitamin C to cover the scientific concepts in chapter 2. If you follow Linus Pauling's thinking, 500 milligrams of vitamin C will seem like the "bare bones." Either way, be sure the vitamin-C supplement you buy contains bioflavonoids.

  If you use medication, such as aspirin, aspirin substitutes, or other medications, consider the 500 milligrams of vitamin C as a basic supplement. Likewise if you smoke, work in or commute in a smoky environment, you'll need more vitamin C.

- *Vitamin E:* Much research supports about 100 international units (I.U.) of vitamin E daily. So I think it's logical to start there with supplements. If you work in a smoky environment, drive in traffic, or work around fumes, take as much as 400 I.U. of vitamin E daily.

- *Beta Carotene:* I would like to see a carotene supplement that contains a mixture of carotenoids, such as lycopene and others. Until then, however, I recommend everyone take 10 to 15 milligrams of beta carotene daily. Alternatively, snack on carrots and eat lots of sweet potatoes. If you spend a lot of time in the sun or a smoky environment, an extra 10 milligrams of beta carotene makes sense.

- *Calcium:* You should make sure you get 1,000 milligrams of calcium daily and up to 1,500 milligrams if you're past menopause. You can do it with milk and dairy products or supplements. These days there's no excuse for falling short in calcium.

- *B-Complex:* There are many reasons for taking extra B-complex nutrients—for instance, if you're under a lot of emotional or physical stress or taking medication (birth control pills, aspirin, high blood pressure medication, and so on). You can take as much as four to five times the RDA of these nutrients. They would be expressed as 400 or 500 percent of the RDA on the label. Select a complete B-complex supplement that is balanced with the RDAs of all the B-vitamins. Don't be confused by the number of milligrams listed on the label as they are different for each vitamin. Select your supplement according to the RDA, because that's what counts.

- *Fish Oil (EPA) or Flaxseed Oil:* If you follow the Longevity Diet you can still benefit by taking extra fish oil—up to about 500 milligrams of EPA daily. Or you can put a teaspoon of flaxseed oil on cereal each day or on salad with the dressing. Flaxseed oil is tasteless, odorless, convenient, and inexpensive.

BALANCED DIET

Americans don't eat a balanced diet. I hope that from now on more of us will. Whenever I teach medical students, I like to show them the composition of a balanced diet and explain the concepts you've learned in this book. One student is always sure to ask: "Who eats like that?" I tell them about 10 percent of Americans and show them the following data:

Who Eats A Balanced Diet?

Food	Approximate Percentages of Americans
No fruit	20
No vegetables	27
No fruit or vegetables	7
No salad	20
Salad less than once weekly	60

America's Food Habits

Beef per capita daily	3.5 oz.
Chicken per capita daily	3.2 oz.
Fish per capita daily	0.2 oz.
Who eats a balanced diet?	About 10%

When I speak to a group of teenagers, I love to ask them, "Who here has a salad regularly?" Usually, all the hands go up. Then I point to one individual and ask: "What kind of salad do you eat?" The usual answer: "I get it with my hamburger." That's a tragedy; young people think the garnish with a hamburger is a salad. Let's change that bankrupt notion.

So your doctor is correct. We *can* get what we need from a balanced diet, but we *don't*. The problem is that most of us don't eat a balanced diet. Actually, the doctors' or dieticians' comments are a play on the words "can" and "will."

ETHNIC FOODS

Food in America reflects all the societies, cultures, and ethnic origins of the people. Each food is "Americanized" a little or a lot, depending on availability of ingredients and convenience. But they still carry the spirit of the old country. Therefore, be patient and recognize that my interpretation of ethnic cuisines is tainted by growing up in America.

All the great cuisines of the world have certain flavors that seem to characterize their cooking. These are usually based on a seasoning derived from local sources that was used to flavor a staple, such as rice or wheat. There are some dominant ethnic tastes:

FLAVOR CHARACTERISTICS OF ETHNIC FOODS

Japanese: Soy sauce, sugar, ginger, and saki
Szechuan Chinese: Soy sauce, ginger root, sugar, and vinegar
Cantonese Chinese: Soy sauce, ginger, peanut, sugar, and garlic
Indian: Curry
Iranian: Yogurt with dill and mint
Greek: Lemon, oregano, dill, cinnamon
Italian: Olive oil, tomato, basil, oregano, garlic, thyme
French: Butter, cream, wine, stock from chicken or meat, mustard, cheese, herbs
Jewish: Chicken or goose fat, onions, garlic, salt
Mexican: Tomato, chili peppers, cumin, lime, garlic

LET'S EXPLORE A FEW CUISINES

• *French:* A scarcity of good quality meat and innate parsimoniousness led the French to use meat as a condiment. The result is an increased use of grain and vegetables with sauces that include spices, onions, garlic, and mustards. While the dish is often rich, its origins were not.

In America, French cuisine is much higher in fat than the French originally intended. So opt for fish, poultry, and game, such as rabbit, rather than beef. The French use of vegetables, especially onions and cruciferous vegetables, is legend. For dessert, poached fruit and fruit tarts are excellent and surprisingly low in calories if not sauced or custardy.

• *Chinese:* Lack of fuel and protein, nutritional need, and poor quality water were the driving forces behind Chinese food. By putting a small amount of meat over a lot of rice, they stretched the quality of their protein. They saved fuel by cooking in a wok, which concentrates the heat better than a flat surface. Vegetables cooked quickly in hot oil preserved nourishment. By using onions, garlic, and cruciferous vegetables, the Chinese have avoided many illnesses. Growing conditions in many parts of China yielded several crops of cabbage annually, allowing it to be abundantly used.

In other areas of China, spicy food protected people from water-borne parasites. Hot spices, especially hot peppers, contain materials that research has shown are effective vermifuges; that is, they kill water-borne parasites that can cause dysentery. This was especially important in areas where human excrement was used as fertilizer in agriculture. And spicy food is common to hot climates. Consequently, spicy Szechuan cooking makes extensive use of spices such as chili peppers. It also emphasizes garlic and onions, with the ubiquitous cabbage and broccoli. Each area of China gives rise to specific foods.

When you eat Chinese foods, select those that feature fish, ginger, garlic, and plum sauces, with special emphasis on vegetable dishes. Chinese vegetable variety and preparations are almost endless. When you eat sweet and sour foods, think of them as an effective means of providing the calcium needs for women and children. Reflect that people have eaten them for ten thousand years.

• *Mexican:* A true vegetarian cuisine that blended corn, beans, and squash to get enough protein of good quality. Add the tortilla, an edible utensil made from corn, with a liberal dash of ground limestone, and you've got a very healthy meal. Hot peppers and other spices prevented intestinal infection for the same reasons it worked in China. These hot spicy foods have stood the test of time.

Two pluses for Mexicans are their abundance of fruit and fish. In our Americanized Mexican restaurants, we seldom see the fruit and fish of true Mexican cuisine. Their fish isn't surpassed anywhere else in the world. Mexicans apply the same spices and cooking techniques to fish as they do to all foods.

Approach Mexican food as if you were a vegetarian. Try to go without meat. You will find that there are no better protector foods available anywhere. Add fish to your menu and the options are endless. Mexicans have so many varieties of vegetables and methods of cooking them that you would never have to serve the same dish twice. You would never run out of Mexican dishes to order in restaurants all over Mexico.

• *Italian:* Another protector cuisine. Italian sauces make use of garlic, onions, carrots, and frequently tomatoes. These sauces are a treasure trove of carotenoids and natural bulbs. In addition, the Italian use of broccoli, beans, and radishes gives them an edge on all the protectors.

The abundant fish near the coast and poultry and rabbit from inland areas provided protein that especially the southern Italians used with tomato sauce. Consequently, their protein sources are low in saturated fat and rich in protectors. Additionally, their generous use of olive oil in southern Italy contributes to such a low incidence of heart disease that it's called the "Mediterranean" experience.

No Italian meal can be complete without cheese. Much Italian cheese, such as ricotta and mozzarella, is low in fat. Fruit and cheese is a dessert or a social snack in Italian homes. Cannolis (pastries filled with ricotta cheese, chips of chocolate, and candied fruit) are one of the best desserts, as they provide calcium, protein, and a modicum of bioflavonoids.

Italy provides excellent soil for fruit, and no Italian table could be complete without a bowl containing pears, apples, oranges, and grapes.

When eating or cooking Italian, think vegetarian. You'll be amazed at the various methods of preparing dishes with pasta, vegetables, several kinds of cheese, and a wide variety of sauces. Then include fish, poultry, or rabbit on your menus. Once more, you can soar through so many dishes that a lifetime isn't enough to either prepare them or eat them in the many restaurants that abound.

• *Greek:* It's unfair to try and separate Greek from Italian cuisine and vice versa, although the Greek climate is different enough to produce other vegetable varieties. Goat cheese is frequently used in Greece. It gives salads a unique flavor. Similar to southern Italian cooking, the Greeks use olives, olive oil, and the cruciferous vegetables. Fish dishes, radishes, fruit, and raw vegetables are also popular.

Try to avoid Greek recipes that call for a lot of meat. Rather, let cheese, especially feta cheese, be the protein source, and you may discover a wonderful, new taste experience. Greek dishes that use eggplant have a unique flavor from their generous use of olive oil, spices, and feta cheese.

EXPLORE

Although this exploration of ethnic foods is by no means complete, you can see that each one can be a protective treasure. The best way to explore ethnic foods is to purchase a cookbook that specializes in a specific cuisine. Read the recipes and search for vegetable dishes. Ask yourself if the fish and poultry recipes use these protein sources as a condiment for staples, such as rice and pasta. If they do, they are probably less American and more authentic. If the sauces are generous with garlic, onions, and ginger, you've got a winner.

APPENDIX

Additional Reading

This reading list is not an exhaustive compilation of the sources used in this book. Rather, it emphasizes review articles, symposium publications, and a few papers that are especially pertinent. The papers cited will get any serious student started in any medical library on discoveries that are rewarding, although never ending.

FOOD COMPOSITION

Bowes and Church's Food Values of Portions Commonly Used. 15th ed. 1989. Revised by Jean A. T. Pennington. Philadelphia: Lippincott.

INTRODUCTION AND GENERAL SOURCES

Alabaster, Oliver. 1985. *The Power of Prevention.* New York: Simon & Schuster.

Committee on Diet, Nutrition, and Cancer. "Diet, Nutrition, and Cancer." 1982. Washington, D.C.: National Academy Press.

Davis, D. L. "Natural Anticarcinogens, Carcinogens and Changing Patterns in Cancer: Some Speculation." 1990. *Environmental Research* 50(2): 322–40.

Doll, Sir Richard. "Symposium on Diet and Cancer: An Overview of the Epidemiological Evidence Linking Diet and Cancer." 1990. *Proceedings of the Nutrition Society* 49(2): 119–31.

Dormandy, T. L. "Free-Radical Pathology and Medicine." 1989. *J. Royal Coll. Physicians of London* 23(4): 221–27.

Essman, W. B., ed. 1987. *Nutrients and Brain Function.* New York: Karger.

Farb, P., and G. Armelagos. 1980. *Consuming Passions.* Boston: Houghton Mifflin.

Finley, J. W., and D. E. Schwass, eds. "Xenobiotic Metabolism: Nutritional Effects." 1985. Washington, D.C.: American Chemical Society.

Food and Nutrition Board of the National Academy of Sciences. 1989. *Recommended Dietary Allowances.* 10th ed. Washington, D.C.

Garn, S. M., and W. R. Leonard. "What Did Our Ancestors Eat?" 1989. *Nutrition Reviews* 47(11): 337–45.

Halliwell, B. "Tell Me About Free Radicals, Doctor." 1989. *J. Royal Soc. Med.* 82(12): 747–52.

Hooker, Richard J. 1981. *Food and Drink in America.* Indianapolis: Bobbs-Merrill.

"Proceedings of the Third Intl. Conf. on the Prevention of Human Cancer." 1989. *Preventive Medicine* 18(5): 553–739.

Scala, James. 1985. *Making The Vitamin Connection*. New York: Harper & Row.

_____. 1987. *The Arthritis Relief Diet*. New York: NAL.

_____. 1988. *The High Blood Pressure Relief Diet*. New York: NAL.

_____. 1990. *Eating Right for a Bad Gut*. New York: NAL.

Schneider, A., and K. Shah. "The Role of Vitamins in the Etiology of Cervical Neoplasia: An Epidemiologial Review." 1989. *Arch. Gyn. and Obstetrics* 246(1): 1–13.

Spiller, Gene A., and James Scala, eds. 1989. *New Protective Roles for Selected Nutrients*. New York: Alan R. Liss.

CHAPTER ONE

Bendich, A., and J. A. Olson. "Biological Actions of Carotenoids." 1989. *FASEB J.* 3(8): 1927–32.

Potischman, N., et al. "Breast Cancer and Dietary Plasma Concentrations of Carotenoids and Vitamin A." 1990. *Am. J. Clin. Nutr.* 52(5): 909–15.

Willett, W. C. "Vitamin A and Lung Cancer." 1990. *Nutrition Reviews* 48(5): 201–11.

Ziegler, R. G. "A Review of Epidemiologic Evidence That Carotenoids Reduce the Risk of Cancer." 1989. *J. Nutr.* 119: 116–22.

CHAPTER TWO

Gey, K. F., G. B. Brubacher, and H. B. Stahelin. "Plasma Levels of Antioxidant Vitamins in Relation to Ischemic Heart Disease and Cancer." 1987. *Am. J. Clin. Nutr.* 45: 1368–77.

Prasad, K. N., and J. Edwards-Prasad. "Expression of Some Cancer Risk Factors and Their Modifications by Vitamins." 1990. *J. Am. Coll. Nutr.* 9(1): 28–34.

Taylor, A. "Associations Between Nutrition and Cataract." 1989. *Nutrition Reviews* 47(8): 225–34.

CHAPTER THREE

Bendich, A., and L. J. Machlin. "Safety of Oral Intake of Vitamin E." 1988. *Am. J. Clin. Nutr.* 48: 612–19.

Chuong, C. J., E. B. Dawson, and E. R. Smith. "Vitamin E Levels in Premenstrual Syndrome." 1990. *Am. J. Obstetrics and Gynecology* 163(5) part 1: 1591–95.

Howard, L. J. "The Neurologic Syndrome of Vitamin-E Deficiency." 1990. *Nutrition Reviews* 48(4): 169–76.

Lloyd, J. K. "The Importance of Vitamin E in Human Nutrition." 1990. *Acta. Paediatrica Scandinavia* 79(1): 6–11.

Smith, S. M. "Vitamin E Lives Up to Its Image as Protective Nutrient." 1989. *Environmental Nutrition* 12(1): 1–2.

CHAPTER FOUR

Fan, A. M., and K. W. Kizer. "Selenium, Nutritional, Toxicological and Clinical Aspects." 1990. *Western J. Med.* 153(2): 160–67.

CHAPTER FIVE

Kendler, B. S. "Taurine: An Overview of its Role in Preventive Medicine." 1989. *Preventive Medicine* 18(1): 79–100.

CHAPTER SIX

Rose, D. P. "Dietary Fiber and Breast Cancer." 1990. *Nutrition and Cancer* 13(1 and 2): 1–8.

Trock, B., E. Lanca, and J. Greenwald. "Dietary Fiber, Vegetables and Colon Cancer." 1990. *Natl. Cancer Inst.* 82(8): 650–61.

Willett, W. C., et al. "Relation of Meat, Fat and Fiber Intake to the Risk of Colon Cancer in a Prospective Study Among Women." 1990. *New England J. Medicine* 323(24): 1664–72.

CHAPTER SEVEN

Spiller, G. A., ed. *CRC Handbook of Dietary Fiber in Human Nutrition.* 1986. Boca Raton, CRC Press.

CHAPTER EIGHT

Cave, William T., Jr. "Dietary n-3 (W-3) Polyunsaturated Fatty Acid Effects on Animal Tumorigenesis." 1991. *FASEB J.* 5(8): 2160–67.

Cohen, M. M., ed. *Biological Protection with Prostaglandins.* 1985. Boca Raton: CRC Press.

Dupont, J., et al. "Food Uses and Health Effects of Corn Oil." 1990. *J. Am. Coll. Nutr.* 9(5): 438–70.

Dyerberg, J. "The Eskimo Experience." 1986. *n-3 News* 1(1): 1–4.

Enig, M., et al. "Isomeric Trans Fatty Acids in the U.S. Diet." 1990. *J. Am. Coll. Nutr.* 9(5): 471–86.

Hwang, D. "Essential Fatty Acids and Immune Response." 1989. *FASEB J.* 3(9): 2052–61.

Isseroff, R. R. "Fish Again for Dinner! The Role of Fish and Other Dietary Oils in the Therapy of Skin Disease." 1988. *J. American Academy of Dermatology* 19(6): 1073–80.

Salmon, J. A. "The Effects of n-3 Fatty Acids on Inflammation." 1987. *n-3 News* 2(3): 1–3.

Simopoulos, A. P., R. R. Kifer, and R. E. Martin, eds. *Health Effects of Polyunsaturated Fatty Acids in Seafoods.* 1986. New York: Academic Press.

Turini, M. E., K. B. Tapan, and M. T. Clandinin. "Prostaglandins-Diet-Cancer." 1990. *Nutrition Research* 10 (7): 819–27.

Wan, J. M-F, M. P. Haw, and G. L. Blackburn. "The Interaction Between Nutrition and Inflammation: An Overview." 1989. *Proc. Nutr. Soc.* 48(3): 315–35.

CHAPTER NINE

Horrobin, David F. "Cardiovascular and Inflammatory Diseases: Interactions Between M-6 and M-3 Essential Fatty Acids (EFAS)." 1990. *Omega-3 News* V(3): 1–6.

Kendler, B. S. "Gamma-Linolenic Acid: Physiological Effects and Potential Medical Applications." 1987. *J. Appl. Nutr.* 39(2): 79–93.

CHAPTER TEN

Bailey, L. B. "The Role of Folate in Human Nutrition." 1990. *Nutrition Today* 25(5): 12–18.

Maso, J. R. "Folate, Colitis, Dysplasia and Cancer." 1989. *Nutrition Reviews* 47(10): 314–17.

Milunsky, A., et al. "Multivitamin/Folic Acid Supplementation in Early Pregnancy Reduces the Prevalence of Neural Tube Defects." 1989. *JAMA* 262(20): 2847–52.

Rosenberg, I. H. "Folate Absorption: Clinical Questions and Metabolic Answers." 1990. *Am. J. Clin. Nutr.* 51(4): 531–34.

CHAPTER TWELVE

Gallager, J. C. "The Pathogenesis of Osteoporosis." 1990. *Bone and Mineral* 9(3): 215–27.

Matkovic, V. "Factors That Influence Peak Bone Mass Formation." 1990. *Am. J. Clin. Nutr.* 52(5): 878–88.

CHAPTER THIRTEEN

Block, Eric. "The Chemistry of Garlic and Onions." 1985. *Scientific American* 252(3): 114–19.

"Proceedings of the First World Congress on the Health Significance of Garlic and Garlic Constituents." In press. Contact: Robert I. Lin, Nutrition International Co., 6 Silverfern Drive, Irvine, CA 92715.

Richardson, Rosamond. 1982. *The Little Garlic Book*. New York: St. Martin's Press.

Sumiyoshi, H., and M. J. Wargovich. "Garlic (Allium Sativum): A Review of its Relationship to Cancer." 1989. *Asia Pacific J. Pharmacology* 4: 133–40.

CHAPTER FOURTEEN

Hocman, G. "Prevention of Cancer: Vegetables and Plants." 1989. *Comp. Biochem. Physiol.* 93(2): 201–12.

Le Marchand, L., et al. "Vegetable Consumption and Lung Cancer Risk." 1989. *J. Natl. Cancer Inst.* 81(15): 1158–64.

CHAPTER FIFTEEN

The Surgeon General's Report on Nutrition and Health. 1988. U.S. Dept. of Health and Human Services, Public Health Service. Publication number 88–50210.

CHAPTER SIXTEEN

Hinman, B., and M. Snyder. *More Lean and Luscious*. 1988. Rocklin: Prima Publishing & Communications.

Read, M. H. "Health Beliefs and Supplement Use." 1989. *J. Am. Dietetic Assoc.* 89(12): 1812–13.

INDEX

A

Adrenal glands, 42, 43, 224
Aerodigestive organs, 26, 27,
    31, 48–49, 70, 77
Age pigment, 69, 70
Age spots, 65, 66, 69
Aging, 65, 123
    and Longevity Diet, 245–46
    and vitamin E, 65, 66, 70,
    78, 82
AIDS, 2
Air sacs, 74, 75
Alcohol, 8, 97, 205, 206, 220
Alcoholism, 73, 104
Alfalfa, 21, 127
Allergies, 60, 230
Allicin, 220–21, 226–27, 230
Alpha linolenic acid (ALA),
    152–53, 162, 165
Alpha tocopherol, 46, 68, 250

American diet, 164, 271–72
Amino acids, 4, 97, 102, 106,
    182–83
    sulfur, 99
Anemia, 67, 182, 183, 190
Antibacterial (antibiotic), 216,
    219–23
Anticonvulsant, 184, 189, 192
Anti-inflammatory, 173, 174,
    179, 189, 192
Antioxidants, 15–107
    in cruciferous vegetables, 237,
    239
    defined, 15–16, 28
Antixenobiotics, 102–3
Appendicitis, 112, 118, 120–
    21
Arachidonic acid (AA), 153,
    162, 174, 175, 177
Arterial plaque, 43, 80, 124–25,
    169

Arthritis, 3, 9, 87, 88, 149,
    158, 169–70, 254
Arthritis Relief Diet, The, 170
Aspirin, 189, 192, 225–26, 269,
    270
Asthma, 149, 158–59, 169, 216
Atopic eczema, 179
Attention deficit disorder, 179
Autoimmune diseases, 158, 159,
    160, 179
Aveolar fluid, 75
Azulfidine, 189

B

Balanced diet, 270–71
B-complex vitamins, 37, 181,
    192, 194, 195, 196–97, 270
Beans, 106, 112, 114, 135, 152,
    193, 199, 216, 273, 274
    and Longevity Diet, 246, 247,
    249
Beef, 7, 150, 248
Beta carotene, 3, 17–39, 66, 74,
    92, 167, 239
    amounts needed, 22, 23, 25,
    35–37, 250, 253
    and cancer, 26–28, 31–35
    and Longevity Diet, 270
    as sunscreen, 23–26
Betel nuts, 29
Bile, 98, 106, 125
    -acids, 124, 207–08, 210
Bioflavonoids, 42, 56, 57, 61,
    253, 274
    and Longevity Diet, 249
Birth control pills, 187, 188,
    189, 192, 270
Birth defects, 182, 184–86, 190,
    192–93, 195, 241

Bladder, 31, 49
    cancer, 9, 17, 22, 27, 31–32,
    36, 49
Blood
    cells, 24, 149
    clotting, 81, 161, 171, 223–26
    fat, 156
    leakage, 67
    pressure, 163, 203, 207, 222–
    24, 254, 255–56
    sugar, 216, 218, 228–29
    testing, 76–77
    vessels, 149, 223
    See also High blood pressure;
    Leukocytes; Platelets; Red
    blood cells
Bones, 203–08
    brittleness, 9, 10, 204
    marrow, 42, 183
Bowel disorders, xiv, 118, 159
Bowel movements, 111, 120,
    129, 132, 135–36, 255
*Bowes & Church's Food Values
    of Portions Commonly
    Used,* 248
Brain, 1, 73, 99, 100, 101–2,
    105, 148, 151, 164–66, 196
    hemorrhage, 67
    tumors, 50, 59, 165
Breast, 78–79
    cancer, xiv, 5, 8, 9, 10, 27,
    41, 49, 50–51, 77, 91, 92,
    129, 149, 159, 160–61, 163,
    235, 240, 253
    milk, 148, 165, 209
Breastfeeding, 94, 97, 148, 175–
    76, 209
Bronchial problems, 66, 75,
    168, 234
Bruising, 43, 224
Bubonic plague, 219, 221–22

Burkitt, Dr. Dennis, 116–23,
124, 125, 126, 127, 130
Burkitt's lymphoma, 116–17
B vitamins, 3, 37, 181, 192,
194, 195, 196–97, 270. *See
also* Folic acid; Niacin;
Thiamin

C

Caffeine, 205
Calcium, 58, 102, 200–14, 270
and cancer, 207, 208, 210
deficiency, 203–08, 209, 210
and Longevity Diet, 270
Calcium carbonate, 206
Calcium oxalate, 58
Calcium phosphorus ratio, 205–
06
Calorie, 116, 136, 138, 267–68
Cancer, xiii, 204, 243, 245, 257
beta carotene and, 26–29
and calcium, 207, 208, 210
and cell division errors, 109
and cruciferous vegetables,
235, 236, 237, 240
and essential oils, 149, 159,
160–61, 163
and fiber, 117–18, 126–29,
130
and folic acid, 186–89, 190
garlic and, 226–27
and heredity, 8
initiator, 44
and niacin, 195, 198
prevention, xiv, 2, 3, 13, 16,
22
and selenium, 89, 91–93
and taurine, 103
vegetables that prevent, 216

and vitamin C, 43, 44–45,
48–51, 55
and vitamin E, 66, 70, 75–78,
82
Canthaxanthine, 18, 20, 30
Capillaries, 67, 74
Carbohydrate, 115, 116, 117
Carbon dioxide, 19, 34, 74
Carbon monoxide, 19, 34
Carcinogens, 26, 91–92, 227
Cardiomyopathy, 89
Cardiovascular disease, 103
Carotenoids, xiv, 1, 17–38, 49,
57, 92, 237, 239, 253
amount needed, 35–37, 250,
270
and cancer, 227
and Longevity Diet, 249
Cataracts, 9, 10, 16, 33, 41, 51,
55, 66, 73–74, 82, 241
Cell, 20, 66, 238
membranes, 19, 20, 34, 45–
46, 70–72, 76, 91, 102, 103
nuclei, 19, 20, 29, 70
reproduction, 183–84
Cellulose, 113, 114, 116
Central nervous system, 42, 43,
69, 70, 72–73, 94, 184
Cereal, xv, 128–29, 132, 134,
199
fiber content chart, 139–40
with insoluble fiber, 114
and Longevity Diet, 246, 249
with selenium, 96
with vitamin E, 84
Cervical cancer, 9, 10, 26, 49
Cervix, 31
Cheese, 201, 213, 214, 247, 274
Chicken. *See* Poultry
Children, 4, 21, 50, 59, 82, 87,
89, 90, 100, 101–2, 117,

Children, *(continued)*
    133, 148, 166, 179, 182,
    194, 221, 256
Chinese food, 272–73
Chlorides, 103
Chlorinated drinking water, 31,
    188
Chlorine, 19
Chlorophyll, 18, 19
Cholera, 220
Cholesterol, xv, 33, 80, 104,
    106, 112, 124–25, 134–36,
    144, 155, 156, 197, 201,
    208, 209, 249, 255, 256
    -lowering drugs, 189, 192
Circulatory system, 254, 257
Cleft lip, 182, 184, 185–86
Cleft palate, 182, 185–86
Clot, 223–24. *See* Blood
    clotting
Codex Ebers, 217, 219, 226
Coffee, 206
Colds, 6, 47, 60, 218, 221, 234
Colitis, 117, 126, 158, 188
Colon cancer, 2, 7, 9, 10, 26,
    49, 91, 92, 112, 117, 118,
    126–29, 188, 207, 235, 240
Colostomy, 128
Congestive heart failure, 103
Constipation, 5, 128
Cooking, 36–37, 42, 48, 177–
    78, 191
Cooper's Disease, 78
Corn, 68, 113, 152, 196, 201,
    273
    bran, 114, 249
    oil, 150, 151, 166, 171
Cornea, 21
Crohn's disease, 149, 158, 188
Cruciferous vegetables, 215–16,
    233–41, 249, 253, 274

Cysteine, 99
Cystic fibrosis, 97
Cystic fibrosis steatorrhea, 103

D

Dairy products, 99, 200, 201,
    212, 213, 214, 270
Degenerative diseases, xiii,
    123
Dementia, 195
Dermatitis, 195, 196, 230
Detoxification, 106, 127,
    129
Diabetes, 100, 131, 149, 158,
    228–29
Diarrhea, 3, 59, 168, 182, 183,
    192, 195
Digestive tract, 3, 24, 98, 112,
    117, 126, 226
Diuretics, 189, 223
Diverticula, 121
Diverticular disease, 112, 115,
    117, 118, 121–23
DNA, 183, 195, 197–98
Docosahexaenoic acid (DHA),
    1, 148, 151, 153, 162, 164–
    66, 169, 170, 171
Dyerberg, Jorn, 154–61, 162,
    170
Dysenteria, 220, 273
Dysplasia (dysplastic cells), 28–
    29, 31–32, 44, 78, 127,
    186–87, 189, 190, 195, 210

E

Eating Right for a Bad Gut, 142
Eicosapentaenoic acid (EPA), 4,

151, 153, 162, 165, 166, 167, 169–70, 171, 225, 270
Emphysema, 3, 9, 11, 33–34, 66, 74–75, 82, 216, 240
Enteric infections, 220
Enzymes, 112, 238–40
Epidemiology, 6–7, 8, 30, 31, 48, 49, 92, 154, 225, 227, 235
Epilepsy, 97, 105, 158, 161
Epithelial tissue, 31, 92
Erythema, 24
Esophagus, 26
cancer, 9, 11, 17, 18, 26, 27, 77, 92, 235, 240
Essential oils, 65, 69, 71, 110, 148–72
amount needed, 166–67, 170–71, 179
and cancer, 159, 160–61, 163
and illness, 157–60, 163, 174
Estrogen, 204
Evening primrose, 173, 174, 177, 178
Excretory organs, 3
Exercise, xv, 81, 200, 205, 206, 253, 255, 256–58
Eye, 1, 21, 73–74, 98, 99, 101, 148, 151, 164–65, 184
lens, 42, 74

F

Fats, xv, 7, 54, 76, 79, 91, 92, 115, 116, 124, 129, 138, 155, 207, 224, 238, 255, 256
absorption, 103, 106
in American diet, 164
defined, 150–51

and Longevity Diet, 249
See also Essential oils
Fetus, 59, 184
Fiber, xiv, xv, 7, 106, 111–31, 134
amount needed, 113, 123, 133, 136–37, 250, 253
and cancer, 126–29, 130
deficiency, 115, 117–27, 129–31
and Longevity Diet, 249, 255, 256
matrix, 37, 113
sources, 112–13, 114, 115, 116, 129–30, 132–47
Fibrin, 224, 225
Fibrocystic breast disease, 67, 78–79, 80
Fish, 1, 41, 85, 106, 115, 151–52, 153, 156, 159–61, 163–68
as brain food, 148, 164–65
and cancer, 160–61
and Longevity Diet, 247, 248, 249
Fish oil, 4, 151, 159, 167, 170, 171, 211, 225, 270
Fish oil supplements, 168–71
Flaxseed oil, 166, 168–69, 171, 248, 270
Folic acid, 110, 181–93, 195
and cancer, 186–89, 190
deficiency, 182–86, 188, 189, 190
and Longevity Diet, 249
Free radicals, 188, 197, 237, 238, 241
and carotinoids, 19, 20, 23, 26, 28, 34
defined, 45–46
and selenium, 90–91

Free radicals, *(continued)*
  and vitamin C, 46–47
  and vitamin E, 66, 69, 70–74
French food, 272–73
Fruit, xv, 13, 18, 112, 130, 134
  with carotenoids, 30, 38
  fiber in, 135, 141
  and Longevity Diet, 246, 249
  with Vitamin C, 41, 57, 59,
    61–63
  with vitamin E, 85

G

Galactose, 41
Gall bladder, xv, 98, 106, 112,
  125
Gallstones, xv, 9, 11, 97, 104,
  106, 112, 124, 125
Gamma linolenic acid (GLA),
  153–54, 162, 173–80
Garlic, 215, 216, 217–32, 273,
  275
  and Longevity Diet, 247
  tablets, 231
Gastrointestinal cancers, 17, 26
Gingivitis, 52. *See also* Gums,
  bleeding
Glucose, 19, 41, 228
Glutamic acid, 99, 181
Glutathione, 46, 90, 93
Gout, 59
Grains, 115, 130, 134, 193, 199
  and essential oils, 152
  and fiber, 114, 137, 143
  and Longevity Diet, 246–47,
    249
  and selenium, 96
  and vitamin E, 85
Greenlanders, 154–60, 161, 225

Green vegetables, 44, 67, 181,
  182, 191, 213, 246
Gums, 114, 115, 134
  bleeding, 43, 52–53, 55, 60

H

HDL cholesterol, 80, 82, 112
Headaches, 183, 222, 226
Heart, 100, 101, 102
Heart attack, 223–26
Heart disease, xiii, xv, 2, 43,
  80–81, 103, 124–25, 130,
  157, 158, 161, 163, 222,
  223–26, 243, 244, 255,
  256, 257
Hemicellulose, 115
Hemoglobin, 34, 183, 229
Hemorrhoids, 9, 11, 112, 115,
  117, 118, 120, 240
Hepatitis, 97, 104
Herpes simplex, 220
High blood pressure, 2, 9, 11,
  90, 149, 207, 210, 216, 218,
  222–23, 255, 257
High blood pressure medication,
  192, 270
*High Blood Pressure Relief Diet,
  The,* 256
Hormones, 79, 100, 110, 129,
  188, 203–04
Hypothyroidism, primary, 158–
  59

I

IBD. *See* Inflammatory bowel
  disease
Ileitis, 188
Immune system, xiv, 3, 9, 11,

21, 47–48, 76, 90, 93, 126, 149, 160, 175, 183
Impotence, 9, 11
Indian food, 272
Indole, 236, 239
Infants, 1, 98, 99, 101, 165, 166, 175
Inflammation, 3, 90, 149, 163
Inflammatory bowel disease (IBD), 9, 11, 126, 141, 159, 168, 170, 188
Inflammatory diseases, 3, 149, 158, 163, 165
Influenza, 221
Insulin, 149, 228, 229
Intestines, 21, 24, 31, 106, 112, 120–21, 207, 210
    cancer, 18, 127, 128, 208
    disorders, 118, 120, 126, 130, 183, 222, 228, 240
Iranian food, 272
Iron, 99, 229
Italian foods, 272, 274

J

Jewish food, 272

K

Kaschin-Beck disease, 88, 89, 90, 165
Keratinized tissue, 21, 24
Kidney, 42, 223
    failure, 9, 11, 222
    stones, 9, 11, 58
Killer cells (Pac-man cells), 160, 163

L

Leeks, 215, 217, 230, 247
Leukocytes (white blood cells), 42, 43, 47, 48, 160
Leukotrienes, 162, 163, 170
Light, sensitivity to, 24–25, 229
Limestone, 196, 200, 201
Linoleic acid, 152, 153, 162, 166, 174, 176, 177, 178
Linolenic acid. See Alpha linolenic acid (ALA)
Linseed oil, 248
Lip, 70
    cancer, 29, 77
Lipofuscin, 65, 69
Liver, 22, 98, 100, 106, 124, 125
    dysfunction, 9, 12, 89–90, 104
Longevity Diet, xv–xvi, 45, 51, 56, 59, 94, 96, 106, 129, 150, 164, 165, 171, 190, 193, 199, 206, 243–58
    menus, 259–75
Low-back pain, 201
Lung, 2–3, 24, 31, 33–34, 47, 70, 74–75
    cancer, 1, 9, 12, 17, 18, 26, 27, 33, 49, 77, 92, 235, 240
Lutein, 30
Lycopene, 16, 17, 18, 20, 22, 30, 31, 36, 49, 250, 270
Lymphatic system, 124

M

Manic depression, 174, 179
Mathews-Roth, Dr. Micheline, 25, 37, 229
Measles, 221

Meat, 42, 85, 99, 101, 106, 163, 175, 199, 205, 206
  and Longevity Diet, 247, 249
Medication, 192, 269, 270
Megoblastic anemia, 190
Melanin, 211
Membranes, 2-3, 24, 45
Memory loss, 9, 12, 69
Menopause, 204
Mental condition, 68, 104, 178-79, 195, 196-97, 257
  depression, 3, 195
  retardation, 165, 184
Metabolism, 4, 31, 43, 196-97, 254, 256
Metamucil, 144
Methotrexate, 189
Mexican food, 272, 273-74
Micronucleated cells, 29
Migraine headache, 9, 12, 149
Milk, 41, 201, 204, 206, 207, 209, 212, 213, 270
  and Longevity Diet, 247
Minerals, 194, 248
Monounsaturated fat, 150, 155
Mother's milk, 1, 98, 99, 175-76
Mouth, 112
  cancer, 17, 18, 26, 27, 29, 48, 70, 77, 92
Multiple sclerosis, 158, 169, 179
Multivitamin-mineral supplement, 96, 192, 193, 252
Muscles, 42, 100, 203, 207, 210
Muscular dystrophy, 67
Muscular weakness, 89, 90
Myotonic dystrophy, 104

N

Nails, 93
National Academy of Sciences Food
  and Nutrition Board, 4, 5, 36, 68
Nerve
  cells, 66, 69, 70, 72-73, 100-102, 105, 203, 207, 210
  disorders, 93
Neural tube defect, 184-85, 186
Neuropathy, 68, 72-73, 179
Niacin, 194-99
  and cancer, 198
  deficiency, 195-97, 216
Night vision, 20-21
Nitrates, 44-45, 48, 54-55, 60, 76, 103, 251
Nitrogen oxides, 19, 47, 74
Nitrosamines, 44-45, 54-55, 76, 227
Nutrition
  as slow-motion tonic, 253-55
  and teamwork, 46, 47, 92, 134
Nuts, 152, 153, 172, 199
  and Longevity Diet, 249
  with vitamin E, 83

O

Oatmeal, 113, 114, 134, 249
Old wives' tales, 1, 17, 18, 31, 219, 228
Olive oil, 150, 166, 171, 248, 274
Omega-3, 66, 71, 110, 126, 151-72
  chart of sources, 168
  in garlic, 225

and Longevity Diet, 248
supplements, 169–71
Omega-6 oils, 71, 110, 151,
    152–67, 171
    sources, 174
Onions, 215, 220, 222, 226,
    228–30, 272, 273, 275
    and Longevity Diet, 246, 247
Osteoarthritis, 173
Osteomalacia, 209
Osteoporosis, 203–06
Oxalic acid, 58
Oxides, 197
Oxidizing agents, 23, 26, 33, 46
Oxygen, 15, 19, 34, 103

P

Pancreas, 228
Pancreatic cancer, 8, 235
Para-aminobenzoic acid, 181
Parasites, 228, 273
Pathogenic bacteria, 220, 221
Pauling, Linus, 58, 269
Peanut oil, 171, 248
Pectins, 115, 116
Pellagra, 195–96, 216
Periodontal disease, 9, 12, 209
Peristalsis, 121, 126
Phenol, 236
Phosphate, 102, 205
Phosphorus, 148, 205–06
Photosynthesis, 19
Pineal gland, 99, 100, 101
Pituitary gland, 42, 43, 99, 100,
    101
Placenta, 100
Platelets, 224
    aggregation, 224, 225
Pleurisy, 234

Pliny, 228
Polyps, xiv, 112, 127–29, 134
Polyunsaturated fats (PUFA),
    155, 166, 171, 248
    defined, 150
    selenium and, 91
    vitamin E and, 66, 69, 70,
    71, 72
    See also Essential oils
Porphyria, 23, 25, 229
Potassium, 102, 223, 256
Poultry, 85, 175, 199, 205
    and Longevity Diet, 247
Preconception, 192–93
Pregnancy, 50, 59, 89, 94, 100,
    165, 183–86, 192–93, 209
Premature aging, 9, 12
Premature infants, 81
Premenopausal women, 50
Premenstrual syndrome (PMS),
    79, 82, 173, 176–78
Prevention
    challenge of, 9–12
    as goal, xiii–xv, 2
    food as, 215–16, 227, 235
    responsibility for, 13
    tomatoes and, 31–32
Processed foods, 111, 152, 177
    meat, 41, 44, 54, 56, 60, 66,
    248
Prostaglandin, 90, 93, 149–50,
    151, 160, 162–63, 174–79
Prostate, 149
Protein, 101–02, 106, 115, 183,
    194
    and Longevity Diet, 247–48
Psoriasis, 149, 158, 169
Psyllium, 127, 135, 144
Pteridine, 181
Pteroylglutamic acid, 181
Pycnogenol, 57

R

Radiation, 46
Raynaud's syndrome, 174, 179
RDA (Recommended Daily
    Allowances), 4–5
  beta carotene, 23, 35
  B vitamins, 270
  calcium, 202, 207
  folic acid, 190
  and Longevity Diet, 249–51
  selenium, 88, 90, 94
  vitamin C, 52, 53
  vitamin E, 68, 81, 82
Rebound scurvy, 58
*Recommended Dietary
    Allowances,* 68, 81
Rectal cancer, 26, 49, 112
Red blood cells, 34, 67, 109,
    162, 183, 186–87
Red fruits and vegetables, 31,
    36, 38, 246
Regulators, 109–214
Reproductive organs, 3
Reservoir, 53–54, 190, 203
  charge, 102
Respiratory problems, 55, 60
Retina, 73, 98, 99, 101
Retinoic acid, 103
Retinol equivalents (RE), 36–37
Rheumatoid arthritis, 87, 88,
    163, 179
Rickets, 209, 210
Risks, defined, 6–7

S

Safflower oil, 150
Salad, 166, 171, 248
Saliva, 48, 49
Salivary glands, 43

Saturated fats, 155, 177, 210
  defined, 150
Schizophrenia, 174, 178
Scleroderma, 9, 12, 169
Scurvy, 40–43, 48, 57, 73
Seed oils, 68, 83, 152, 153
Selenium, 16, 46, 77, 87–96,
    165
  amount needed, 88–90, 94,
    253
  safety, 88, 90, 94
  toxicity, 93–94
  and vitamin E, 66, 71, 89–90,
    91–92, 94
Shallots, 215, 221, 230, 247
Side effects, 180
  of beta carotene, 23
  of EPA, 169–70, 171
  of garlic, 223, 226, 230
  of niacin, 197
Sjogren's syndrome, 179
Skin, 9, 12, 31, 245
  anatomy, 24
  cancer, 2, 9, 12, 17, 18, 26,
    27, 33, 92, 211, 235
  color, 23, 24, 25, 33, 210
  disorders, 2, 23, 24–25
  sensitive and dry, 18
Smoked meats, 44, 54, 60
Smoking, 7, 8, 18, 26, 31, 33–
    34, 46, 56, 66, 74–75, 161,
    185, 187, 188, 205, 224,
    255, 269
Snuff dipper, 29, 31
Sodium, 102
Sperm agglutination (clumping),
    52, 55
Spicy food, 273
Spina bifida, 182, 184
Spleen, 42
Staphylococcus, 220

Steatorrhea, 103
Steroids, 31
Stomach, xiv, 49, 112
Stomach cancer, 26, 77, 92,
    227, 235, 240
Stool, 113, 117, 119, 121, 126,
    135–36, 182
Stress, 126, 158, 224, 270
    and vitamin C, 41, 47, 48, 54,
    55, 56, 60
Stroke, xiii, xv, 149, 158, 161,
    216, 223–25
Sugar, 124, 178, 194
Sulfasalazine, 188
Sunlight (sunshine), 17, 18, 19,
    25, 33, 41, 56, 195, 229
    and beta carotene, 22–
    25
    and vitamin D, 208–11,
    250
Superoxides, 19, 20, 26, 28, 46,
    70, 90–91, 103, 188, 238,
    239
Superoxide dismutase, 239
Supplement, xvi
    B-complex, 270
    calcium, 206, 207, 212, 213,
    270
    carotenoid, 37, 270
    fiber, 132, 135, 136, 143–44,
    146
    fish oil, 168–70, 171, 172,
    248, 270
    folic acid, 185, 186, 188, 189,
    191–92
    garlic, 231
    GLA, 179–80
    and Longevity Diet, 249,
    269–70
    megadoses, 252–53
    need for, 251–53

selenium, 96
    vitamin C, 51, 59–60, 269
    vitamin E, 86, 269
Sweet and sour cooking, 201,
    273
Swollen joints, 43
Synergistic effect, 71, 74,
    90

T

Taurine, 4, 97–107
    and cancer, 103
    deficiency, 98
Testes, 42
Testicles, 52, 67, 116
Thiamine, 3
Thiocynate, 234, 236
Throat cancer, 18, 26, 27, 29,
    48, 70
Thromboxanes, 163
Thyroid toxicosis, 159
Tocopherol, 65, 67, 68,
    250
Tocotrienols, 68
Tomato, 17, 18, 20, 22, 30, 31–
    32, 36, 59, 246, 272, 274
Tongue, 183
Toxicity
    of selenium, 93–94
    of vitamin A, 22, 23, 250
    of vitamin D, 33, 211, 250
Toxins, xiv, 19, 20, 24, 25, 31,
    103, 126, 127, 222, 240,
    250, 251
Trace mineral, 88
Tranquilizers, 192
Tumor development, 70, 75–76,
    78, 161, 226–27
Typhus, 220

U

Ulcer, 159, 240
Ulcerative colitis, 118, 126, 170, 188
Ultraviolet (UV) light, 2, 4, 20, 26, 33, 46, 209, 211, 251
Uric acid, 59
Urine, 31, 54, 103
Uterus, 31, 187

V

Vagina, 31, 149
Vaginitis, 220
Varicose veins, 112
Vegetables, xiv, xv, 13, 17, 112, 115, 130, 134, 163
  with calcium, 213, 214
  with carotenoids, 30, 36, 37–38
  cooked vs. raw, 36–37
  fiber in, 114, 135, 142–43
  folic acid in, 191
  and Longevity Diet, 246, 248–49
  and vitamin C, 57, 59, 63–64
  and vitamin E, 68, 85
  See also specific types
Vermifuge, 228, 273
Vision loss, 66, 222
Visual sensitivity, 9, 12, 66, 68, 73
Vitamin A, 3, 17, 20–22, 29, 36
  amount needed, 22, 35
  toxicity, 22, 23, 250
Vitamin C, xiv, 5, 6, 16, 37, 40–64, 76, 165, 237
  amount needed, 42–43, 45, 51, 52–56, 58–61, 250, 253
  and bioflavonoids, 57

and cancer, 43–45, 48–51
deficiency, 40, 43, 47, 48
and free radicals, 46–47
and illnesses other than cancer, 51–55
and Longevity Diet, 249, 269
and selenium, 93
and vitamin E, 66, 71, 73–74, 78
Vitamin D, 33, 200, 208–12
  and cancer, 208
  toxicity, 33, 211, 250
Vitamin E, 16, 46–47, 51, 57, 65–86, 174, 237, 239, 250
  and aging, 65–68, 69–70
  and cancer, 75–78
  deficiency, 67–68, 73, 81
  and illnesses other than cancer, 72–75, 78–81
  and Longevity Diet, 249, 269–70
  and selenium, 71, 89–92, 94
  and vitamin C, 66, 71, 73–74, 78
Vitamin K, 81
Vitamins, 3–5. See also specific vitamins

W

Water, 44, 54, 58, 60, 102, 113, 115, 188, 228
  balance, 100, 102
  and Longevity Diet, 248
Weight, xv, 5, 7, 98, 192, 222, 228, 245, 255–56
Wheat, 68, 112, 113
  bran, 114, 122, 127, 134, 249
  fiber, hard, 128
  germ, 65

White blood cells. *See*
  Leukocytes
Women, 41, 79, 202–07

X

Xenobiotics, 102–03

Y

Yeast
  brewer's, 194, 199
  infections, 220
Yellow vegetables, 18, 30
Yogurt, 201, 206, 213, 214
  and Longevity Diet, 247